Seven Steps to Managing Your Aging Memory

Seven Steps
to Managing Your
Aging Memory

What's Normal, What's Not, and What to Do
About It

Second edition

ANDREW E. BUDSON, MD
Neurology Service, Section of Cognitive & Behavioral Neurology and
Center for Translational Cognitive Neuroscience
Veterans Affairs Boston Healthcare System
Alzheimer's Disease Research Center & Department of Neurology
Boston University School of Medicine
Division of Cognitive & Behavioral Neurology, Department of Neurology
Brigham and Women's Hospital
Harvard Medical School
Boston, MA
Boston Center for Memory
Newton, MA

MAUREEN K. O'CONNOR, PSYD
Psychology Service, Section of Neuropsychology,
Bedford Veterans Affairs Hospital
Bedford, MA
Alzheimer's Disease Research Center, Department of Neurology
Boston University School of Medicine
Boston, MA

OXFORD
UNIVERSITY PRESS

OXFORD
UNIVERSITY PRESS

Oxford University Press is a department of the University of Oxford. It furthers
the University's objective of excellence in research, scholarship, and education
by publishing worldwide. Oxford is a registered trade mark of Oxford University
Press in the UK and certain other countries.

Published in the United States of America by Oxford University Press
198 Madison Avenue, New York, NY 10016, United States of America.

Library of Congress Cataloging-in-Publication Data
Names: Budson, Andrew E., author. | O'Connor, Maureen K., author.
Title: Seven steps to managing your aging memory: what's normal, what's not, and what
to do about it /by Andrew E. Budson, MD and Maureen K. O'Connor, PsyD
Description: New York, NY : Oxford University Press, 2023. | Includes bibliographical
references and index.
Identifiers: LCCN 2016042463 | ISBN 9780197632420 (hardback)
Subjects: LCSH: Memory disorders—Treatment. | Memory. | BISAC: MEDICAL /
Neurology.
Classification: LCC RC394. M46 B83 2017 | DDC 616.8/3—dc23
LC record available at https://lccn.loc.gov/2016042463

DOI: 10.1093/oso/9780197632420.001.0001

This material is not intended to be, and should not be considered, a substitute for
medical or other professional advice. Treatment for the conditions described in this
material is highly dependent on the individual circumstances. And, while this material is
designed to offer accurate information with respect to the subject matter covered
and to be current as of the time it was written, research and knowledge about medical
and health issues is constantly evolving and dose schedules for medications are being
revised continually, with new side effects recognized and accounted for regularly. Readers
must therefore always check the product information and clinical procedures with the
most up-to-date published product information and data sheets provided by
the manufacturers and the most recent codes of conduct and safety regulation. The
publisher and the authors make no representations or warranties to readers, express
or implied, as to the accuracy or completeness of this material. Without limiting the
foregoing, the publisher and the authors make no representations or warranties as to the
accuracy or efficacy of the drug dosages mentioned in the material. The authors and the
publisher do not accept, and expressly disclaim, any responsibility for any liability, loss,
or risk that may be claimed or incurred as a consequence of the use and/or application
of any of the contents of this material.

Printed by Sheridan Books, Inc., United States of America

Contents

STEP 7   PLAN YOUR FUTURE

Preface

- You walk into a room to get something and forget why.
- You cannot think of the name of a friend at church even though you have met her a half-dozen times.
- You cannot remember as many details of important events of your life as your spouse, including those such as your wedding and family vacations.
- A week after seeing a movie you have trouble remembering the name of the movie and parts of the plot.
- When you are driving and not paying attention, you take one or more wrong turns and end up somewhere you didn't intend to be.
- You cannot come back with the correct items from the store unless you write them down and look at the list.
- You spend too much time looking for your keys, glasses, wallet, or purse.
- You find yourself having difficulty finding your car in a parking lot.
- You find yourself looking at the calendar multiple times a day to remember your schedule.
- Your family tells you that you've asked that question before.

Do some of these experiences sound familiar?

Do you find it difficult to know which of these experiences are likely due to normal aging and which are likely due to a memory disorder?

Do you sometimes have these or other memory problems?

Do you joke that you have "senior moments" or suffer from "CRS" (frequently translated as "can't remember stuff")?

Have you ever wondered—or worried—whether a slip of memory could indicate the start of Alzheimer's disease?

Do you want to have your memory evaluated but are not sure how to go about it?

Are you nervous about what the evaluation will consist of and what will and will not be covered by Medicare or other insurance?

Would you be interested in taking a medication if it would actually improve your memory?

Are you interested in helping your memory with healthy foods and diets but confused by all the conflicting claims?

Would you like to know whether doing crossword puzzles or playing computer games can improve your memory and stave off Alzheimer's disease?

Do you want to start exercising to help your memory but are not sure what is the right type or amount of exercise to do?

Have you been diagnosed with mild cognitive impairment?

Have you been diagnosed with Alzheimer's disease?

If you answered "yes" to any of these questions, this book was written for you. We can help you with your memory. We can explain which lapses of memory are normal and which are not. We can teach you diets and exercises that can help. We can provide you with strategies and activities to improve your memory and keep it strong. And we can help you know when you should see your doctor and what your doctor should do about your memory problems.

In our practices as a neurologist and a neuropsychologist, we have evaluated several thousand individuals with concerns about their memories, just like you. We help them understand when their memory difficulties are due to normal aging, vitamin deficiencies, or depression and when they are due to diseases such as Alzheimer's. Depending upon the cause of the problem, we then recommend particular medications, vitamins, diets, exercises, or group activities, and sometimes even clinical trials of new medications being developed.

So why now and why this book? When we are discussing the results of these evaluations and our recommendations with individuals, we often wish that we had more time—more time to explain our rationale as to why their memory problems are likely due to normal aging versus a serious disorder, more time to explain how and why a medication works, and more time to explain the pros and cons of various treatments and recommendations. This book provides us with the opportunity to tell you all of the information about these and other topics, from which you can take in as little or as much detail as you would like.

Why a second edition? Although you may feel worried about having memory problems, today there is more we can do to diagnose and treat memory problems than ever before. In just the last few years there has been an explosion of new diagnostic tests and criteria to help evaluate memory loss, as well as a huge expansion in our knowledge of treatments, diets, and exercises to help memory in individuals aging normally as well as in those with mild cognitive impairment, dementia, and Alzheimer's disease. The US Food and Drug Administration (FDA) has approved both amyloid and tau brain scans, meaning that the plaques and tangles that cause Alzheimer's disease can now be visualized in the living brain. And since the first edition, blood tests to diagnose Alzheimer's are now available, and the first medication for Alzheimer's that has the potential to slow down the course of the disease has been approved by the FDA. There are also new studies that help us understand the influence of sleep, alcohol, and cannabis on the brain. This book is our opportunity to share these advances with you and help you manage your memory in seven basic steps.

Why does this second edition emphasize that it is *Seven Steps to Managing Your Aging Memory*? We wanted to clarify that this book has been written specifically for you—an older individual who wants to know if their aging memory is normal or not and, either way, what to do to keep their memory as strong as possible. Since the first edition of this book, we have now published a book specifically for family members (and other caregivers) whose loved one has Alzheimer's disease or another dementia, as well as a book that explains the science behind normal memory and how to use that knowledge to remember better. See the *How to Use This Book* section for more on these new books.

Acknowledgments

The genesis of this book began with the excellent questions posed to us by individuals with memory concerns and their families. We would therefore like to begin by thanking them for the inspiration and guidance they have given us. Next, we would like to thank our friends and family members who read various drafts of the first edition of this book and provided their invaluable feedback: Fred Dalzell, David Wolk, Jeanie Goddard, Amy Null, George Null, Richard Budson, Sandra Budson, Leah Budson, Adnan Khan, Brigid Dwyer, Kate Turk, Cecilia McVey, Peter Grinspoon, Suzanne Gordon, Barbara Wojcik, Nan Pechenik, Susan Fink, and Barbara Mindel; we couldn't have done it without you. An additional special thanks goes out to Dennis O'Connor and Todd Harrington for their support. We are also grateful to our colleagues and mentors who have taught us so much about caring for individuals with memory concerns, including Paul Solomon, Elizabeth Vassey, Kirk Daffner, Dan Press, David LaPorte, Michael Franzen, Keith Hawkins, Richard Delaney, Patricia Boyle, Malissa Kraft, Lee Ashendorf, Helen Denison, and Edith Kaplan. Finally, a big thanks to our editor, Craig Panner, who saw our vision, had the courage to encourage us, and guided and supported us through the process.

The content of this book has been derived from the patients whom the authors have seen in their private practices along with literature reviews conducted solely for the purpose of this book. These reviews and the writing of this book have been conducted during early mornings, late nights, weekends, and vacations. Their contribution to this book was conducted outside of both their VA tours of duty and their Boston University/ NIH research time.

How to Use This Book

We set out to write this book to be as useful to as many people as possible. If you are:

- *An older individual with concerns about your memory*, this book was written with you in mind. We suggest that you read the book cover to cover.
- *A family member (or friend) of someone whom you are concerned about*, this book was also written for you. We suggest that you read the book cover to cover as well.
- *An older individual without any memory problems or concerns, but with a desire to strengthen your memory*, we suggest that you read Steps 1, 2, 5, and 6. Other Steps can be read if you wish.
- *An individual of any age who wishes to learn more about memory, including late-life memory disorders, their treatments, and the diets, exercise, and strategies that can help*, please read any Steps you wish.
- *A healthcare professional*, this book can be recommended to your patients to help them better understand memory, memory disorders, their treatments, and the diets, exercise, and strategies that they can do to manage their memory.
- *An educator*, this book can be used as an easy-to-read text on memory and memory disorders, full of case examples.

- *A family member (or other caregiver) whose loved one is in the moderate to severe stage of dementia,* this is not the right book for you. We would suggest our book *Six Steps to Managing Alzheimer's Disease and Dementia: A Guide for Families* by Andrew E. Budson and Maureen K O'Connor.
- *A student who hopes to use this book to improve their performance on exams,* this is not the right book for you. We would suggest *Why We Forget and How to Remember Better: The Science Behind Memory* by Andrew E. Budson and Elizabeth A. Kensinger.

About the Stories

To make this book more accessible, we have woven stories throughout the text. As we mention later, we hope that these stories will make it easier to understand the issues we are discussing and their implications. If, however, you would prefer to read the text without the stories, please do so. You can skip them altogether, or you can read specific stories when you want more information on a particular topic. We've written the book so that the stories are optional. To make it easier to jump into the stories in the middle, we've included the cast of characters below.

Sue, an eighty-year-old woman with concerns about her memory
John, Sue's husband
Jack, a seventy-two-year-old man with concerns about his memory
Sara, Jack's daughter
Sam, a mutual friend of both Sue and Jack. Sam's wife, Mary, has Alzheimer's disease.

Introduction

That could have been embarrassing, Sue thinks to herself. She was halfway through lunch with one of her closest friends, before the name of her friend's husband came to her. *How could I have forgotten?* she thinks again. She is able to remember everything about him—what he looked like, his career as a surgeon, his retirement party—except his name.

Sue was able to cover for this little memory lapse. In fact, she has become quite good at covering for memory lapses, such as trouble coming up with someone's name, and laughing it off when the lapse was noticed. Sue herself, however, isn't laughing.

Sue is worried about her memory. Worried, in fact, is a bit of an understatement. She is absolutely terrified that she is developing Alzheimer's disease. She just turned eighty, the same age that one of her friends, Mary, was diagnosed with this disease. Since that time Mary has had to move out of her apartment and into a facility.

Sue hasn't mentioned her concerns to her friends or her children. Her children would only worry and overreact—wanting her to go into one of those "retirement communities." She doesn't need that . . . after all, she has no difficulty living in her home. She does her own shopping, cooking, and cleaning, and she has never been late with a bill payment. Her friends wouldn't be interested in hearing about her concerns. It would only make them anxious about their own, similar memory difficulties—or

worse, they would start to treat her like an invalid and stop
including her in their social activities. She has mentioned her
concerns to her husband, John. He doesn't think her memory
is abnormal, and she doesn't want to worry him by bringing it
up again.

Sue thinks about some of her other memory lapses. Just yesterday she walked downstairs to the basement and could not
remember for the life of her what she was looking for. It was
only when she walked back up to the kitchen that she remembered the roll of paper towels that she needed, which she then
successfully walked down to get. She doesn't have trouble
remembering things that happened yesterday or last week, but
she finds it quite difficult to recall some of the things from her
childhood, such as the name of her best friend in second grade.
Is that normal? Sue isn't sure.

Sue is having trouble remembering names, walking into a
room and not knowing why she is there, and recalling some
of the information from her childhood. Yet she is completely
independent with everything she does in life—and she wants to
stay that way. She is quite concerned about her memory. Should
Sue be worried?

Let's consider another story. Jack has just come from his
local community lodge where Sam, one of his buddies, suggested that Jack get his memory checked out because Sam
thought Jack could be developing Alzheimer's disease or
dementia.

Could he be right? Jack thinks about Sam's words. He isn't sure
whether he should thank Sam—or slug him. Part of him wants
to do both. Deep down he knows that Sam is trying to be helpful, but he has a lot of nerve. Sure, Jack knows he has some
trouble remembering, but who his age doesn't? Just because
Sam's wife has dementia, all of a sudden he thinks he's a god-
damn doctor. Not that the doctors know very much about
memory problems, from what Jack could tell. Sam had to take

Mary to her doctor four times before the doctor actually did anything about it.

Jack considers his memory. He didn't think anything was wrong, at least, not any more than with anyone his age. He is seventy-two, after all. Sure, his memory isn't as good as when he was thirty-two (or sixty-two, for that matter). At least half his friends—maybe three-quarters of them—have similar difficulties coming up with people's names and remembering the details of what they did yesterday or were going to do the next day. The more he thinks about it, the more he thinks his memory is probably normal . . . better than normal, in fact. How many people his age can list off their buddies from high school and the make, model, and year of the cars that they drove? Heck, he can even remember some of his friends from grade school. Jack appreciates that he doesn't know very much about dementia or Alzheimer's disease, but he'd bet that few people his age can remember details of their childhood like he could.

Still, Jack feels unsettled. Sam stressed that the reason he was bringing it up was because there were medications Jack could take that would improve his memory. He doesn't want to be stupid—he had seen his neighbor ignore his high blood pressure and then suffer a stroke that left him unable to talk. Sticking his head in the sand is definitely not the right thing to do. After all, he has never been one to run away from a problem; he'd rather stand and confront it. Perhaps he should call his doctor.

Do the stories of Sue or Jack sound familiar? We will be following Sue and Jack throughout this book to illustrate the seven steps to managing your aging memory. We will be with them as they gain a better understanding of normal memory (Step 1) and, partnering with their doctor, get a thorough evaluation (Step 2). We'll watch as various disorders are considered and a diagnosis is made (Step 3). We will see the medications they are prescribed (Step 4), the diets, exercise regimes, and other lifestyle factors they explore (Step 5), and the habits, strategies, and aids they use to improve their memories (Step 6). We'll also see them struggle with issues of mood, anxiety, and adjustments in their lives that need to be made. Finally, we'll see where they turn for additional resources and how they plan their future (Step 7).

We hope that these stories—composites of real people we have worked with—will make it easier to understand the issues we are discussing and their implications. If, however, you would prefer to read the text without the stories, please do so. We've written the book so that the stories are optional.

Without further ado, we now turn to Step 1 to understand normal memory and the changes in thinking and memory associated with healthy aging.

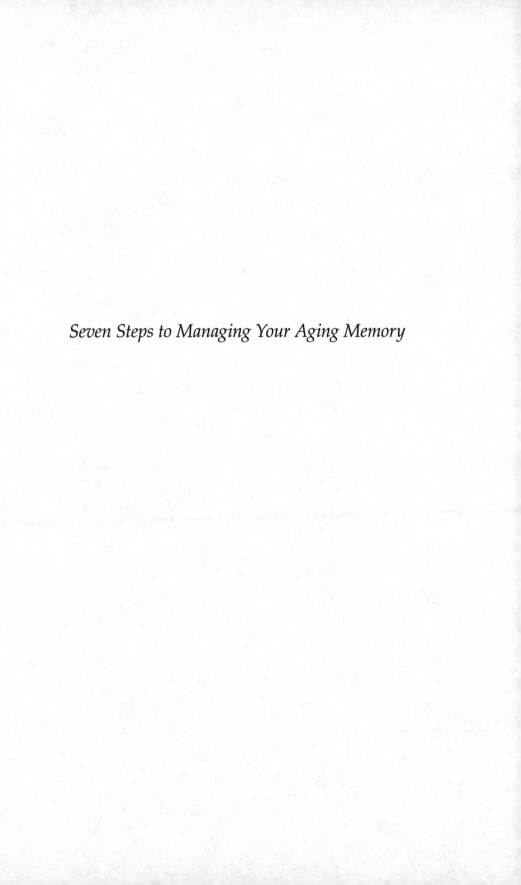

Seven Steps to Managing Your Aging Memory

Step 1

LEARN WHAT IS NORMAL MEMORY

Is your memory normal? To answer that question we need to start with a different question: What is normal memory?

In Step 1 we will learn about the problems that are part of normal memory. One thing that makes memory loss tricky, however, is that the difference between normal and abnormal memory isn't necessarily the type of problems that occur but rather the frequency and severity of those problems. Nonetheless, in order for us to begin to help you know if your memory is normal or not, we need to first tell you about the memory errors that can happen to anyone of any age and then let you know what changes occur to memory as we get older.

1

Which Memory Errors Can Happen to Anyone of Any Age?

In this chapter we will take a look at a number of different ways that memory often fails in healthy individuals of any age, leading to forgetting or even distorted and false memories. We'll also begin to explain how memories are formed, stored, and retrieved.

MEMORIES FILL UP THE PAGES OF OUR LIVES

Sue (whom we met in the Introduction) and her husband, John, are visiting Washington, DC, for the first time since they took their children there about forty years ago. They are excited to see which parts of the city have remained the same and which have changed. Although she hasn't mentioned it to John, Sue is also using this visit to test her memory—to see what she can and cannot remember of their prior visit. They are eating lunch at the Garden Café in the National Gallery of Art.

When we speak about memory, in general we are referring to memory for the episodes of our lives. Think about an episode of your life, such as the last lunch you had with a friend. The episode would include the sights of the restaurant and your friend, the sound of your friend's voice, and the smells and tastes of the foods, as well as your thoughts and feelings at that time. When you are creating a memory, the information from your senses, thoughts, and emotions becomes drawn together in a coherent story, just as if you were writing it down. Each separate sensation—say, the sound of your friend's voice—would constitute an aspect of the memory. The different aspects would come together to represent the several parts of the episode. For example, one part could be your impressions of the waiter: what he looked like, including his clothing, haircut, mannerisms, and voice. Another part would be what drink you ordered, whether a glass of water, diet soda, or cocktail with a little umbrella in it. There would be a part for your lunch entrée, and a part for what your friend ordered. There would be parts for your conversation—different parts for each topic you discussed.

THE HIPPOCAMPUS BINDS THE MEMORY TOGETHER

When the episode is over (in this case when your lunch is over), the different aspects of each part of the event and the different parts themselves become bound together as a coherent whole: a memory. Once the episode is bound it can then be stored so you can later retrieve it as a whole. In fact, once bound together, thinking about any part of the memory, such as your entrée— or even the smell of your entrée—can bring the entire episode to mind. The binding is coordinated by the hippocampus, the memory center of your brain. There's one on each side, left and right. They are located deep inside your brain on the inside and bottom of each temporal lobe, which are next to your temples on each side of your head, just behind your eyes. The left hippocampus is somewhat specialized for remembering verbal and factual information, and the right for nonverbal and emotional information.

MEMORIES FADE WITH TIME

After lunch, Sue and John walk across the grassy National Mall to visit the National Air and Space Museum.

"I'm really looking forward to seeing what the Air and Space Museum looks like now compared to how it was when we were here with the kids," John says as his shoes crunch along the gravel path.

"Are you sure that we visited this museum?" asks Sue. "I don't recall having been to it before."

"Yes! I'm absolutely sure. I have a vivid memory of it because we were here on the bicentennial—1976—and it had just opened. You know how interested I was in space then."

"I know we were here in DC on the bicentennial, I just don't recall going inside the Air and Space Museum."

They walk through the door of the museum, enjoying the cool air inside.

Sue looks up and sees the *Spirit of St. Louis*, the Lunar Module, and several other air and space craft. She is now quite sure that John is right, and that she has been in the museum before. She can recall vividly how it felt to be standing under the *Spirit of St. Louis* forty years ago. "John," she says, "you're absolutely right. I now remember being here and seeing these hanging planes and spaceships."

Sue pales slightly as she thinks about having forgotten that she was in this museum before.

Memory is transient; things we remember don't tend to stick around forever. There is a gradient in which events that occurred recently are relatively easier to remember than events that occurred in the more distant past. There are many myths about memory, and one of them is that we are supposed to remember everything that ever happened to us, particularly if it was notable, even if it happened long ago. Thus, you may worry if you cannot remember details of that notable vacation you took to Great Britain twenty years ago. However, not remembering details of a vacation from many years ago may be perfectly normal, particularly if you haven't thought about that vacation much over the years. When you think about a memory, it is as if you are re-experiencing and then re-storing the memory again, so it stays fresh and easy to recall. But a memory that doesn't get thought about at all will fade with time. How quickly will it fade? It depends on how strongly the memory is formed in the first place. The more unusual the episode—such as meeting the Queen of England—the stronger the memory will be and the longer it will take for the memory to fade. In later chapters we'll consider other factors that also help determine how strong a memory is when it is formed.

Now let's turn to one of the most common reasons that memories fail.

YOU NEED TO PAY ATTENTION TO FORM A MEMORY

After spending several hours enjoying the Air and Space Museum, Sue and John stroll west along the gravel path of the Mall, past some of the other Smithsonian buildings. Finally they reach their destination, the World War II Memorial, which is new since they were last here.

"Hey Sue, listen to this," John says as he reads from a plaque. "Freedom Wall holds 4,048 gold stars. Each gold star represents 100 American service personnel who died or remain missing in the war. The 405,399 American dead and missing from World War II are second only to the loss of more than 620,000 Americans during our Civil War . . ."

Sue isn't really listening. She has noticed a family that reminds her of their family when they were younger. *The father, trying to teach the children some history. The girl, hanging on every word. The older boy, interested, but trying not to look too interested, because he needs to look "cool." The mother, trying to keep the younger boy from making a run for it . . .*

They continue exploring the monument, making a slow loop around its large grounds.

When they have explored for about a quarter of an hour, Sue notices a wall filled with brass stars. "What do you think," she asks John, "are these stars just here for decoration or do you think that they mean something?"

"I read you the explanation about fifteen minutes ago."

"You did?" Sue asks with surprise.

"Yes. Each star represents 100 American service men and women who died or went missing in the war."

"Oh . . . OK, thanks. I must have forgotten."

Oh no, not another thing I am forgetting! Sue thinks to herself as she feels another wave of anxiety flooding through her.

Not paying enough attention is the number-one reason that healthy individuals experience difficulty remembering names, events, and that thing you went into the other room to get. Life is busy. We are often doing two things at once. If you are doing one thing—say, responding to an email—and someone interrupts you to ask you to do a few things, it wouldn't be surprising that you might forget one of the things you were asked to do. The reason is that your attention was focused on your email and not on the person who interrupted you and the things you were asked you to do. This situation is an example of not paying attention causing a failure to learn new information.

Thus, when you are introduced to someone and then thirty seconds later—while still talking to him—you cannot remember his name, the problem is caused by the fact that you were not paying enough attention to his name; you were probably busy trying to listen to what he was saying or thinking of what you could say next.

Now let's turn to the second type of not paying attention, that which occurs when retrieving a memory.

YOU NEED TO PAY ATTENTION TO RETRIEVE A MEMORY

After their time at the World War II Memorial, John flags down a cab and he and Sue climb in. John gives the driver the name of their hotel in Georgetown, and the cab begins moving. It is election season, and everyone is talking politics.

"Where are you from?" asks the driver.

Sue tells him, and asks, "Is everyone in this city obsessed with politics?"

"Yes, absolutely," he responds. "Especially when there's an election coming up."

The three of them continue to chat about politics and the impending election.

"Excuse me," John says urgently to the driver, "but are you sure this is the way to Georgetown?"

"You're absolutely right, sir," the driver responds as he turns off the meter. "You got me talking politics and I started driving to the airport automatically, without thinking about it," he says apologetically, as he turns the car around.

When we are carrying out actions automatically and our attention is focused elsewhere, we may not pay enough attention to a memory we are retrieving. Driving "on autopilot" and ending up in the wrong place is common and just one example of what happens when we are preoccupied and not focusing our attention on the information we should be retrieving—in this case information related to where we are supposed to be going.

We can now explain one of the most common failures of memory: when you walk into a room to get something but cannot remember why. What typically happens is that when we walk in to get a particular item, we often see something else that triggers a new and different thought, and we become distracted, lose the focus of our attention, and then cannot remember what we walked in to get. Here we are suffering from not paying enough attention. For example, let's say that we are going from the kitchen to the basement to get a screwdriver to tighten a knob on a cabinet door. We walk down the basement stairs, see the washing machine right in front of us, and remember that we need to finish doing the laundry. This simple thought of remembering that we need to move the clothes from the washer to the dryer distracts us sufficiently so that we temporarily forget about the screwdriver, and now we cannot recall what we went downstairs to get. When we give up trying to remember why we went downstairs and walk back up to the kitchen, we see the open cabinet door in front of us, remember that we need to get the screwdriver, and this time successfully go down to get it.

Let's take a look at another common memory difficulty.

SOMETIMES A NAME IS ON THE TIP OF YOUR TONGUE

"So who are you going to vote for?" asks the driver, now heading for Georgetown.

"I'm going to vote for Governor Jones," John responds.

"And what about you Ma'am, are you voting for Jones, too?"

"Me? No, I'm voting for Senator . . . Senator . . ." Sue says, struggling to bring up the senator's name.

"You mean Senator Smith?" asks the driver. "Yea, he's got my
vote, too. Least bad of the bunch, in my opinion."

Have you ever been at a party and seen someone you know
approaching you from across the room but cannot remember her name? You may remember many things about her—
she lives in your town, has a son and a daughter, works at the
school, and plays golf—but you can't remember her name, even
though you know it and you can almost feel it "on the tip of
your tongue." Good news—it's completely normal. Having a
name "on the tip of your tongue" is the most common example
of blocking—not being able to retrieve information from your
memory even when it is in there.

Sometimes blocking a name occurs because you keep
thinking of a similar but incorrect name. The incorrect name
is "blocking" the right one. That's why if you stop trying to
retrieve the name and think about something else for a while,
the correct name may pop into mind.

Thus far we have examined how memories fail when we are
trying to store or retrieve information. Let's now turn to how
memories can become mixed up, distorted, and outright false.

SUGGESTED INFORMATION CAN BE
TURNED INTO FALSE MEMORIES

The next day Sue and John are planning to visit the Lincoln
Memorial.

"I'm really excited to see it," Sue says as they are getting dressed
in the hotel. "I know I've seen the Lincoln Memorial on TV and
from a distance, like yesterday, but I don't think I've ever been
to it up close, in person. I know it is supposed to be impressive."

"Sue," John begins, "we definitely saw it with the kids on that first
trip. I'm absolutely sure about it. I remember trying to keep their

attention long enough to read them the Gettysburg Address from the wall before they started running all over the place. I think I got about halfway through before I gave up . . . everyone's kids were running around, and it was a losing battle."

Hmm, Sue thinks to herself, *maybe I have been there before . . . I didn't think I was at the Air and Space Museum either, but John was right about that.* She thinks about it more, trying to imagine it, trying to put herself at the memorial. She pictures the white marble walls, colored with age, the children running around, John trying to read the words and teach them something—as he always does. She can start to see herself there, walking slowly up the steps, trying to keep track of the children. She thinks, *Maybe I have been there before . . .*

Sue continues to think about the Lincoln Memorial as they climb into the cab. The more she thinks about it, the more she believes that she has been there before. The scene becomes more vivid and she pictures the location of the wall with the Gettysburg Address, John, their children, and the great seated statue of the man himself. She can picture herself reaching up and putting her small hand on the massive hand of the statue of Lincoln.

"You know, John," Sue begins, "I'm sure you are right, that I did see the Lincoln Memorial with you and the kids."

"Just wait till you're in front of it," John says. "I'm sure the memories will come back to you."

The cab lets them off, and they walk to the steps of the memorial.

Sue walks up the steps, waiting for the memories to come back to her. She reaches the floor level and begins to walk across to the seated statue. Something is wrong. *This view doesn't match my memory,* she says to herself. She continues to walk slowly around the floor of the memorial. She then goes right up to the statue and looks with surprise how large and high up it is. *I could never have touched the hand of the statue.* "John," she says aloud, "Now that I am here I'm quite sure that I have never been here before. The picture I envisioned in my mind is completely different from how it actually looks."

"Really?"

"Yes. Do you think you could have been here without me?"

"You know, now that I think about it, I don't actually remember you here. Maybe that's why it was so hard to keep the kids under control—because you weren't around to corral them!" he says, chuckling.

Think about an attorney questioning a witness by asking "leading" questions. Compare an open-ended request, such as "Describe what happened when you were at the bank," to a leading question, such as "Describe what happened when the defendant stormed into the bank, brandished a revolver, and asked the teller for money?" These suggestions in the leading question make it more likely that the witness will actually remember the defendant storming into the bank, brandishing a revolver, and asking the teller for money. False memories—even highly elaborate and detailed ones—can occur in individuals with normal memory.

In day-to-day life this type of suggestibility occurs in more mundane but often important settings. Asking individuals if they took their medications in a leading way may make them think that they took them when they didn't. When we ask the question: "You took your pills this morning with your breakfast, right?" we are asking the individual to look inside and see if that memory is there. If just a part of the memory is there—for example, eating breakfast—the suggestion that he also took his pills may be all that is needed for him to falsely remember that he took his pills, when in actuality he did not.

MEMORIES CAN BECOME DISTORTED, MIXED UP, OR CONFUSED

That night Sue and John are eating dinner at an elegant French restaurant. Classical music is playing in the background.

"I love this piece by Bach," Sue says. "I think I played this concerto in high school."

"I like Bach, too," John agrees, "but are you sure that this piece is by Bach? I thought this was Handel."

"No, I'm sure it's Bach."

Just then the restaurant manager comes by their table. "How is everything with your dinner this evening?"

"Wonderful," John responds.

"What piece of music is playing?" Sue asks.

"This is Handel's Water Music . . . do you like it?" asks the manager.

"Very much, thanks," Sue responds.

After the manager departs, Sue says, "Oh John, I don't know what's going on with my memory lately . . . I really thought that piece was by Bach."

We generally expect that when we retrieve a memory it will be accurate. It turns out, however, that memories are frequently distorted, mixed up with other memories, or otherwise confused. Have you ever thought that one of your friends told you something but later realized that the information was from a different friend? Mixing up elements of memories is extremely common. One common example of this type of confusion is when you clearly remember that you locked the front door of your house in the morning, but when you return from your errands, you find, to your surprise, it is unlocked. The usual cause of this type of memory mix-up is that you were remembering locking it on another day. Memories of anything that we do frequently can easily be misattributed to the wrong time. Another frequent example is when you think that an idea is your own creation, but you actually learned the idea from a book you had read. Or perhaps you thought about doing something and then later believe that you actually did it, such as sending an email.

We'll finish our examination of the ways that memory can fail in individuals of any age with two other ways that memories can become distorted.

WE TEND TO REMEMBER THE PAST THE WAY WE VIEW THE PRESENT

A few days later, Sue and John are back at home. Sue is in the family room.

John walks in saying, "Hey Sue, look what I found!" He's holding up an old photo album. "Our pictures from Washington, DC, on that trip with the kids."

Sue and John begin to look at the old photographs.

"I can't believe that people used to wear those polyester pants suits . . . no one looked good in those," Sue says.

"Fashions come and go," John remarks.

"Well, I'm glad that I never owned such clothes . . . you wouldn't have caught me dead in one of those pants suits."

The next group of pictures is from the Air and Space Museum. There are many pictures of planes and spaceships.

"Hey, here's one of you," John says. "I knew you were in the Air and Space Museum with us."

"Yes, you were definitely right about that . . ."

Sue isn't thinking about being in the museum; she is looking at what she was wearing.

"John, let me see the album a minute," Sue says as she moves the photo album onto her lap. She flips through page after page. There is no doubt about it. One, two, . . . and three. She was wearing three different polyester pants suits during their trip to DC.

Just then John notices what Sue is looking at. "Hey, you used to wear those pants suits, too!" he remarks.

"Yes, well, I guess we are all caught up in the fashions of our time," Sue says as she thinks to herself with a sinking feeling, *another thing I didn't remember . . .*

We all have a tendency to have a coherent image of ourselves over time. So although we might say, "I was more liberal in my youth until I learned more about how the world really worked," in general, our picture of ourselves and the views we have held in adulthood is more of a stable, unchanging image than a movie showing the evolution of our views over time. In other words, we tend to remember our own attitudes and viewpoints from the past through the lens of the present. These effects tend to be strongest for feelings, emotions, likes, and dislikes. Thus, although we might be unlikely to misremember major factual details of a trip to the Middle East, our memories of how happy we thought the people were may be colored by whether there is turmoil or peace in the Middle East today. Another common example is how we view another person. Let's think of a colleague at work whom we have known for a long time. When we are getting along with him quite well, we may feel that he has always been a great person, and we remember the times he helped us and his important accomplishments. However, our very memory of him can change quickly if, later on, we find ourselves at odds with him. Now when we think of him, we recall all the mistakes he has made and the problems he has caused.

WHEN WE RETRIEVE A MEMORY, WE MAY ACCIDENTALLY CHANGE IT—PERMANENTLY

Earlier in this chapter, we mentioned that whenever we retrieve an old memory, it is as if we are re-experiencing and then re-storing the memory again, so it stays fresh and easy to recall. Although this re-experiencing and then re-storing has the advantage of strengthening the old memory so that it can be more easily retrieved, the disadvantage is that if there are specific parts or aspects of the memory that are, for whatever reason, recalled incorrectly, those incorrect aspects will be stored and become part of the memory. At a later time when we retrieve the memory, it is likely we will recall the memory with the incorrect information now incorporated into it.

Say we watched a movie, perhaps *The Godfather*, with some friends from work. Later, we see the movie again with our spouse. A few years go by and someone asks us if we have seen *The Godfather*. When we recall the memory, we begin to confuse the two times that we have seen the movie together. The next time someone asks us if we have seen *The Godfather*, we think back and respond, "Yes, I saw it with some friends at work, and I think my spouse was there, too," again rewriting the memory. Finally, another year goes by and someone asks us if we have ever seen *The Godfather*, and we respond with confidence, "Yes, I saw it at our house with my spouse and some friends from work."

SUMMARY

Memories for episodes of our lives are bound together by the memory center of the brain, the hippocampus. Memories fade with time but can be strengthened when they are retrieved. Attention is important when forming and retrieving memories. Lastly, memories can easily become mixed up and distorted over time.

Now that we understand these ways in which memory can fail in anyone, let's review some common memory complaints—including some of those we encountered in the Preface and Introduction—and see which aspect of normal memory explains them.

- You walk into a room to get something and forget why.
  - This symptom is a common, normal phenomenon. Not paying enough attention because you become distracted by something you see in the room is typically the cause.

- You cannot think of the name of a friend at church even though you have met her a half-dozen times.
  - Blocking, when you cannot recall something you know on the tip of your tongue, is a frequent phenomenon. It can be entirely normal, particularly for names of people and other proper nouns.
- You cannot remember as many details of important events of your life as your spouse, including those such as your wedding and family vacations.
  - The fact that memories become less accessible over time is a normal part of memory. Whether the forgetting of a specific event is normal or not, however, depends on many factors, including how long ago the event occurred, how important it was to you, and how often (if ever) you thought about it.
- When you are driving and not paying attention, you take one or more wrong turns and end up somewhere you didn't intend to be.
  - Driving on "automatic pilot" and accidentally driving toward where you usually go (work, home, school, etc.) is very common and due to not paying enough attention.
- You can remember the activities that your grandchildren are doing, but you mix them up, thinking that your grandson is playing baseball and your granddaughter is taking karate, when it is actually the other way around.
  - Attributing real memories to an incorrect time, place, or person is the most common cause of mixing up memories like these, and it can be perfectly normal.
- You are quite sure that you never liked Richard Nixon until your spouse finds your old campaign buttons and sign-up sheets in the attic, and then you recall you actually went door to door to sign up voters to get Nixon on the ballot during his first senate campaign.
  - Here is a clear example of how your present knowledge, beliefs, and feelings about Nixon changed your memory of how you felt about him in the past.
- Your partner asks if you left the iron on before your left the house, and although you initially thought you turned it off, the more you think about it the more you think he is right and you left it on. You turn the car around and drive home, only to find that the iron was off all along.

- o Incorporating suggested information provided by others into your own recollections frequently occurs with leading questions. It is a common cause of false and distorted memory.
- You are at a cocktail party when you notice your zipper is broken. Just then the host of the party introduces you to four people you haven't met before. As you continue chatting with them, you realize that you cannot recall any of their names.
  - o Here is another common and completely normal example of forgetting due to not paying attention when forming a memory. Because your attention was partly focused on your zipper, you didn't have enough attention remaining to learn their names.
- You run into an old friend you haven't seen for many years. You ask her if she is still working at the local bookstore and whether online sales have hurt their business. After staring at you with a confused look on her face, she gently reminds you that it is not she but your mutual friend who works at the bookstore.
  - o Although a bit embarrassing, this error is a fairly common and benign example of mixing up memories. Because they are friends, you are more likely to mix up elements of their lives than if there was no connection between them.

By now we hope that you are breathing a sigh or two of relief that at least some of the memory issues you are experiencing may be completely normal. In Chapter 2 we will turn to memory in older adults and examine some other memory problems that are common in healthy aging.

2

How Does Memory Change in Normal Aging?

After considering some of the most common ways that memory fails in healthy individuals of any age, let's now turn to some of the problems that frequently arise as one gets older.

YOUR FRONTAL LOBES ORGANIZE YOUR MEMORIES

When we last saw Jack (whom we met in the Introduction), his buddy Sam had just told him he should get his memory evaluated because Sam worried that Jack was developing Alzheimer's disease or dementia. Let's check in on Jack now.

Jack's granddaughter, eleven years old and in the fifth grade, needs to do a report for social studies. The family computer isn't working, so Jack volunteers to take her to the library to show her "what everyone did before computers."

Jack drives her to the library. The parking lot is almost full, and they need to park in one of the furthest spots from the entrance. "I'm doing a report on continental drift," she tells Jack excitedly as they are parking and walking toward the building. "Did you know that California is going to break off and fall into the ocean one day?" She continues to chat in an unbroken stream as they walk into the library.

About thirty minutes later, Jack and his granddaughter walk out of the library, book in hand. As Jack looks at the parking lot, he pauses and asks half to himself, "Now which way is the car?"

Jack scans the parking lot, does not see his car, and thinks to himself, *Damn, this is one of those memory problems that Sam was talking about!*

"Where did we park the car?" Jack asks his granddaughter.

"Umm, I don't know. . . . I think it was over here," she responds, pointing vaguely toward the left.

Jack looks to the left and thinks, *Well, the kid doesn't know where the car is either, so maybe it's not just me. . . . Still, I shouldn't be losing my car in the stupid parking lot.*

Have you ever wondered how you can keep track of all of the different memories in your head, make new ones, and recall them when you need to (at least most of the time)? It is the part of your brain called the *frontal lobes* that helps you organize your memories. They are located—as you would expect—in the front part of your brain, just behind your forehead. The frontal lobes help you choose exactly what you are paying attention to, which, in turn, determines what you will remember. Think about all the different sights coming in from your eyes, sounds coming in from your ears, tastes and smells from your mouth and nose, and thoughts and emotions arriving from other parts of your brain. It is your frontal lobes that allow you to choose whether to pay attention to the conversation you are having with your friend or where you are parking your car. The information you are paying attention to is then transferred to the hippocampus and bound into a memory (see Chapter 1). It is also the frontal lobes that help you to search for a memory when you need it. So when you are "trying to remember something," such as where you parked your car, it is the frontal lobes that are doing the "trying," searching through your memories for the correct information.

THE FRONTAL LOBES FOCUS ATTENTION

Is it a sign of serious memory problems if you have trouble finding your car in a parking lot? Not necessarily—particularly if you were speaking with a friend, absorbed by the conversation, and not paying attention to where you parked the car. As we learned in Chapter 1, not paying attention when forming memories is one of the most common causes of not remembering something. Now we can understand a bit more of exactly what the problem is: it is your frontal lobes that are not paying attention in a situation like this one. It is also the frontal lobes that need to focus attention when attempting to retrieve a memory.

OLDER FRONTAL LOBES NEED MORE EFFORT TO PAY ATTENTION

After a bit of searching, Jack and his granddaughter find the car and start to drive home.

"Thanks so much for taking me to the library, Grandpa! I really like this book. I think it is going to be great for my social studies report . . ."

She continues talking in a nonstop stream. Upon arriving home, she runs out of the car almost before it stopped in the driveway, and then runs into the kitchen.

"Did you get a good book?" asks Sara, her mother.

"Yes, Mom, look at this one!" she replies, thrusting the book toward her.

"It looks great," says Sara. "Thanks for taking her to library, Dad."

"Are you going to work on your report now?" Sara asks her daughter. "If you are, you should take your Ritalin."

As we get older, our frontal lobes age along with the rest of us, and we are simply not able to pay attention as easily as we did when we were younger. We can, however, pay close attention in many settings—it just takes a bit more effort. It's sort of like our older frontal lobes have attention-deficit/hyperactivity disorder (ADHD). So if you find that you are having increased difficulty paying attention or sustaining attention, making careless mistakes, not following through on activities, having difficulty organizing tasks, losing things, and becoming easily distracted, it may be because your aging frontal lobes are having more difficulty. These difficulties in paying attention may be a normal part of getting older, and they may be causing your memory difficulties in daily life. One way to confirm that your memory problems are due to poor attention is that these memory problems resolve (or become considerably better) when you use more effort to pay close attention to your activities. We'll discuss strategies to improve your attention in Step 6.

STIMULANTS CAN HELP THE FRONTAL LOBES FOCUS AND PAY ATTENTION

Sara gives her daughter her Ritalin and then starts to make a pot of coffee.

"Would you like a cup, Dad?" Sara asks as she pours herself a steaming mug.

"Sure, thanks," Jack responds.

Jack's granddaughter is working on her report on the kitchen table while Jack and Sara are sipping coffee with cream in the living room. "Is that stuff, the Ritalin, really good for her?" Jack asks.

"Well, I hate it that she has to take a pill, but there is no question that it really helps her focus on her work. Without it, she cannot sit still and bounces all over from topic to topic," Sara responds.

"Yes, I know what you mean," Jack says, thinking back to her freewheeling conversations with him earlier that day. "You make a good cup of coffee, Sara, thanks!"

"Thanks, Dad. You know, Ritalin isn't that different from a cup of coffee. Both can make you more alert and help you focus on what you are doing."

"I never thought about it like that," Jack responds, trailing off in thought. "That makes a lot of sense . . . all those late nights on the job, whenever I needed to pay attention, I would drink coffee and then I could focus on my work."

Mild stimulants such as Ritalin can help a child with ADHD be more awake, alert, and focused on a task. When the frontal lobes aren't able to focus our attention, sometimes a bit of a mild stimulant is helpful. Although we don't typically recommend a prescription medication such as Ritalin for an older adult, you may find that a cup of coffee, tea, or other caffeinated beverage can be helpful for enabling your older frontal lobes to pay more attention, which facilitates both forming and retrieving memories. Note that more is not better when it comes to stimulants; if you take too much of them, it just makes you jittery, and your ability to pay attention actually decreases.

OLDER FRONTAL LOBES HAVE MORE DIFFICULTY STORING INFORMATION

"Sara, do you think my memory is OK?" Jack asks, tentatively.

"Oh, I don't know, Dad," Sara replies, "probably, for your age. What makes you ask?"

"Well, you know Sam down at the lodge? His wife has Alzheimer's disease, and so now he's playing doctor and diagnosing everybody with it."

"And he thinks you have Alzheimer's disease?"

"Yeah," Jack sighs, "have it, or could be developing it."

"Well, have you had any trouble remembering things?"

"Sure, but I can't figure out whether it is more than anyone else my age. I didn't think it was, but now Sam has me wondering."

"What sorts of things are you having trouble remembering?"

"Well, you know how I was always on the road going to different customers' houses? I used to be able to just glance at an address, and I would be able to memorize it. Now, any time I need to learn a new address, I need to go over it about ten times before I've got it memorized."

"That doesn't sound so bad. What else are you having trouble remembering?"

"What I'm supposed to be doing. I mean, I put things down on the calendar—like picking up your energetic daughter from soccer practice next Tuesday—and it takes me forever to be able to remember it. I now recheck the calendar all the time to make sure I'm not forgetting something that I'm supposed to be doing."

"Dad, I'd be lost if I didn't use the calendar on my phone to keep track of all of my appointments and her activities!" Sara replies, chuckling.

"Yeah, but you don't understand. I used to be able to look at my schedule of all the jobs I had to do during the day—what needed to be done, the customers' names and addresses—and I would have it memorized for that day. I just can't do that anymore," Jack says with concern.

Is it normal to experience more difficulty learning new information now that you are older compared with when you were younger? It certainly can be. We discussed earlier how our older frontal lobes cannot pay attention and take in new information to be bound in the hippocampus and stored in our memory as easily as when we were younger. Repeating information can help overcome our older frontal lobes' difficulty paying attention. Thus, it may be perfectly normal if you need to go over your shopping list, an address you are driving to, or the day's activities a couple of times in order to remember them. We'll discuss other strategies to improve your attention and memory in Step 6.

OLDER FRONTAL LOBES HAVE MORE DIFFICULTY RETRIEVING INFORMATION

As Sara thinks about how good her father's memory used to be when he was younger, she realizes that he may be right—it may have declined. She is also struck by the concern in his voice.

"OK," Sara says, "I get it, Dad. You're having more trouble learning new information than you used to. Have you noticed any other problems?"

"The other thing that really bugs me is how difficult it is for me to recall people's names," Jack replies. "And I'm not talking about the names of someone I just met, although that is particularly hard. I'm talking about people that I've known forever. Take . . . oh, I still cannot remember his name . . . well, take whatever-his-name-is, my friend from high school, for example. This other guy was telling me about his '64 Chevy Impala, a red, two-door coupe with 425 horsepower, and I wanted to tell him that my buddy from high school had the same car—except it was a convertible in green—and I couldn't for the life of me come up with his name. It was only much later in the conversation when I finally remembered it."

Difficulty recalling names is one of the most common problems that healthy older adults experience. If the difficulty is only in recalling names for people and places (proper nouns) then it is usually normal, as we learned in Chapter 1. The bottom line is that recalling information is typically more difficult as we get older, even when the memory storing that information is intact.

IT IS EASIER TO REMEMBER THINGS YOU KNOW SOMETHING ABOUT

After hearing her father tell this story of the cars in such detail, Sara begins to laugh.

"What's so funny?" Jack asks.

"You are!" Sara responds. "You don't seem to have any trouble remembering things that are important to you—like cars."

Jack pauses, thinking about Sara's point. "Well, I'm sure you're right that I have an easier time remembering things that are important to me, but in this case I think it is because I've paid attention to cars all of my life, so it is easy for me to remember when someone tells me about their car."

We all find it easier to remember things that we already know something about, regardless of our age, such as flowers, recipes, or power tools. Let's say it is cars. When you learn a new bit of information on cars, the memory doesn't need to be created completely from scratch; much of the memory can be stitched together from older memories with just the new bit of information added. One reason that some older adults have difficulty learning how to use a computer or a smartphone is that they have no prior experience with such devices and thus no similar older memories that can be stitched together with just the new bit of information. Instead they need to form completely new memories, which is more difficult with older frontal lobes.

IT IS EASIER TO REMEMBER THINGS THAT ARE IMPORTANT TO YOU

Jack sips his coffee, thinking.

"You know Sara, you're definitely right about my having an easier time remembering things that are important to me,"

Jack says. "I can remember when your daughter was born as if it were yesterday. Although we were waiting for the news, it was still exciting when your mother and I got the call that we had a healthy granddaughter. We were just finishing washing the dishes and I almost dropped the plate I was drying. I will never forget the feeling of holding her in my arms and looking down at that little face, sleeping. You looked very happy . . . tired, but happy. And I remember your mother smiling. It's too bad she isn't with us. She would've loved to see her granddaughter, so happy and healthy, running all over and getting into everything."

There are several reasons why it is easier to remember things that are important to us. One is that most important events are emotional, and we remember events charged with emotion better than nonemotional events. We also tend to think about events that are important to us more than other events, going over the memories in our minds. As we learned in Chapter 1, thinking about the event keeps the memory fresh and easy to retrieve.

IT'S MORE COMMON TO MIX UP MEMORIES AS WE AGE

"Yes, I can remember some things very well," Jack says, returning from his reminiscing to the present. "But other times I get things mixed up! Just last week I went to meet Sam for lunch: I'm waiting for him at the lodge when my cell phone rings and it is Sam, asking where I am. I tell him I'm waiting for him at the lodge, and he tells me he is waiting for me at the diner down the street. I thought he was the one who screwed up, but when I got home, I looked at the calendar and there it was: 'Meet Sam at diner.' I guess that's why Sam's worried about me."

"Have things like that happened a lot, showing up at the wrong place?" Sara asks.

"Yes—wrong place, wrong time—it's been happening more and more. I don't know if it is just part of getting older, but I think I'm going to get it checked out. I'm not going to sit around worrying about it."

We discussed in Chapter 1 how distorted, mixed-up, and outright false memories can happen to anyone of any age. As our frontal lobes age, however, these types of confused and muddled memories become more likely to happen.

SUMMARY

Our frontal lobes help us to pay attention, store and retrieve information, and organize our memories. Older frontal lobes don't work quite as well as they did when they were younger, requiring us to put in more effort to pay attention, learn new information, and recall information or events. Stimulants (such as a cup of coffee) can improve our ability to pay attention. Lastly, it is easier to remember things if we know something about them or if they are important to us.

Let's review some common memory complaints in light of what we have learned about normal memory in the older adult. Because the difference between normal and abnormal memory is often related to the extent of the memory difficulties, we will also note examples of when the memory problems would be considered abnormal.

- You come out of the mall after several hours of shopping, and you have to search for your car in the parking lot before you can find it.
  o Difficulty finding one's car in a parking lot is one of the most common memory failures. One common cause is not paying attention when the memory was being formed—particularly if

you were distracted as you were parking or walking from your car, such as if you were talking to a friend.

o It is not normal to search for your car for over an hour or to need assistance in finding your car.

- Your friend is giving you directions to his house. Although the directions are not overly long or complex, he needs to repeat it to you three times before you can remember it.

o Needing information to be repeated in order to remember it may be normal for anyone of any age. Older adults typically benefit from repetition more than younger adults. So don't worry if you need to review information more than once, whether it be directions, a shopping list, or someone's name.

o It is not normal, however, to quickly forget information once it has been learned well.

- You saw a movie last week that you really enjoyed. You're recommending it to your friend, and you cannot recall the name of the movie until, with effort, you go through a list of possibilities in your mind until you finally get the right name.

o Difficulty retrieving information can certainly be perfectly normal, and it is more common as we get older. Cues that can trigger our memory for the information we are looking for typically help, whether it is an external cue (given to us by another person or the environment) or one that we generate ourselves in our minds.

o It is not normal to fail to recognize information we learned when we are provided with strong cues. So if our friend names the titles of several movies and one of them is the one we saw last week, we should be able to correctly choose it from the list.

- You find yourself looking at the calendar multiple times a day to remember your schedule.

o Assuming you have two, three, or four appointments on your daily calendar, it is perfectly normal to need to look at it a couple times in order to remember it.

o If, on the other hand, you find that you need to look at your schedule many more times than you used to and even then you sometimes get confused and end up in the wrong place or at the wrong time, it is not normal.

- You are looking forward to having lunch with your friend Jackie tomorrow until you look at your calendar and see that it is Joan you are having lunch with tomorrow; you're having lunch with Jackie next week.
  - o It can be perfectly normal to mix up information like who you are having lunch with, and this type of mix-up is more common as one gets older.
  - o It is not normal, however, for the memory confusion to lead you to actually show up at the wrong place or time for an event or to miss an event entirely.
- You're meeting with your gardener to discuss what you and your spouse would like to plant. The gardener names ten different types of plants and asks you which ones you would like. You're about to ask for the list again when your spouse—apparently remembering them all—asks how four of them would look together.
  - o If your spouse is an avid gardener, whereas you couldn't tell a begonia from a rhododendron, it is perfectly normal for him or her to have an easier time remembering a list of plants than you. We all have an easier time remembering information when it is related to things we already know or are expert in.
- You and your friend from Boston watch a baseball game together. Turns out it is the game where the Red Sox clinch the division, beating the Yankees. Although you are an avid baseball fan, you follow the Washington Nationals. Reliving the game afterwards over dinner, you notice that your friend can remember almost every play and at bat, whereas you can only recall a few.
  - o We all have an easier time remembering information when it is important to us. There are few things as important to a Red Sox fan as beating the Yankees and clinching the division, so it is not surprising that our friend, a baseball fan from Boston, remembers the game better than we do.
- After attending a weekly community college course for several months, you notice that you remember the lectures better on the days you have a cup of coffee before class.
  - o Most of us find it easier to pay attention when we have a mild stimulant such as coffee, tea, or a caffeinated soda. When we pay attention better, we also remember better.

- You cannot come back with the correct items from the store unless you write them down and look at the list.
  - Most people need to write grocery items down on a list in order to purchase the correct items. Once you've written the list, however, it mainly acts as a reminder or checklist so that you don't forget an item.
  - If you frequently purchase the wrong items at the store so that you don't come home with the items that you need, or you frequently purchase items you don't need because you don't remember that you already have thirty-four cans of peas in the cupboard, it is not normal.

In Step 1 we discussed the memory problems that are normal in healthy younger and older adults and contrasted some of those memory problems that are normal with memory problems that are abnormal. We are now ready to turn to Step 2 to better understand the memory failures that are not normal, the evaluation that your doctor should do, and when referral to a specialist is needed.

Step 2

DETERMINE IF YOUR MEMORY IS NORMAL

In Step 1 we learned about normal memory, including the memory failures that are common and may be perfectly normal in younger and older adults. In Step 2 we will learn about how to determine whether your memory is normal, including understanding the types of thinking and memory problems that are common in Alzheimer's disease and how to work with your doctor if you are concerned about your memory. We'll also learn about the different parts of an evaluation that are helpful in sorting out memory loss.

3

What Kinds of Memory Problems Are Not Normal?

In this chapter we'll consider some common thinking and memory problems that could be caused by Alzheimer's disease.

After her memory difficulties on her trip to Washington, DC, Sue is more worried than ever that she is developing Alzheimer's disease. Let's catch up with her now as she is speaking with Sam. Sam's wife, Mary, a friend of Sue's, was diagnosed with Alzheimer's disease. They are meeting at the bookstore café in the local mall.

"Thanks for chatting with me, Sam," Sue says. "I'm sure it must be hard for you to talk about Mary's illness."

"Actually, I'm very pleased to talk with you about it," Sam replies. "I feel like I've learned so much about memory loss, Alzheimer's disease, and dementia over the last few years that it makes me want to share what I know with others. And there's so much more that they can do now to diagnose and treat memory loss than just a few years ago—if there is ever a good time to have memory problems, it is now."

"Thanks, Sam, that's encouraging to hear."

"So what do you want to know?"

GETTING LOST MORE FREQUENTLY CAN INDICATE A PROBLEM

"How did it start with Mary? What were some of her initial symptoms?" Sue asks casually, stirring her tea as she tries to hide the nervousness in her voice.

Sam looks closely at Sue, seeing the worry in her eyes. Looking down at his coffee, he then takes in a deep breath and exhales slowly before replying. "Well, everybody's different," he begins, looking back up at Sue, "but I think with Mary it started when she began to get lost while she was driving. Mind you, I didn't know what was going on at first. I just knew that it would often take her a long time to go from one place to another. And she knew it would take her a long time, too—she started leaving the house twenty, thirty minutes—even an hour—earlier than she should have needed to get to an appointment. I understand now that she was leaving earlier so that if she got lost, she would have time to straighten herself out and still get to her appointment on time. Looking back, I also realize that she had begun to drive to fewer places. It was as if the circle of where she would go was getting smaller and smaller. First, she didn't drive into the city. Then she didn't drive anywhere new. Then she didn't want to drive on the highway. I didn't really notice it, or at least I didn't think it was a big deal. I mean, who really wants to fight the traffic in the city or highway anyways? The red flag to me was when I got a call from the doctor's office at two o'clock in the afternoon saying she hadn't shown up for her one o'clock appointment. Now mind you, she had left the house at noon for this appointment, and she should have been able to get there in about twenty minutes. So now I'm starting to get worried: Did she have an accident, was she OK? A few minutes later she comes through the door, in tears, telling me that she couldn't find the doctor's office. You know where the office is, right? I mean, he's your doctor, too, so you know it can be a bit tricky to find. But Mary's been going there for over ten years! That was the thing that made me realize something was really wrong."

Anybody of any age can get lost. You make a wrong turn, things don't look familiar, or you're trying to find a new place and all of a sudden you're lost. Normally, however, you're able to quickly correct your error. You pull over and ask for directions, reset your GPS device, or maybe pull out a map from your glove compartment or your phone. In any event, after a few minutes you're oriented and back on your way.

With Alzheimer's disease, however, once you make a wrong turn it isn't so simple to get back on track. Because memory is impaired, there are few landmarks that look familiar. Because thinking is impaired, maps, GPS devices, and phone apps can be confusing and difficult to use. You can stop for directions, but they are often too long and complicated to remember. It therefore becomes common for those with Alzheimer's to drive to fewer places than they used to. When that happens, the disease is interfering with their ability to be independent, to go where they want to go. The bottom line is that if you are getting lost to the point that it changes where you are comfortable traveling, it is abnormal.

LOSING THINGS MORE OFTEN MAY SUGGEST A PROBLEM

Sue sips her tea as she thinks about Mary getting lost. *Poor thing, it must have been so difficult for her.* "When was that?" Sue asks.

"Oh, must have been five or six years ago, when Mary was seventy-five," Sam responds.

Wow, Sue thinks to herself, *Mary has been struggling longer than I thought.* "I never suspected there were problems so long ago," she says.

"We tried to hide the problems at first," Sam replies simply.

"I thought Alzheimer's was all about memory problems, not getting lost. Did she have any memory problems?"

"Yes," says Sam, setting down his coffee. "Those were probably the next bunch of problems to come up. She was always losing everything in the house. It used to take her forever to get ready—yes, I mean even longer than before—because she was always looking for her glasses, purse, keys, phone. You know . . . looking back now, I think her losing things did happen about the same time as when she was getting lost . . . at the time I just thought she was disorganized."

"Well, she was always a bit disorganized. I bet that didn't help."

"No, it certainly didn't, except as an excuse that I think explained away the problem with losing things to everyone—including me—and maybe even to herself."

Everyone misplaces items from time to time: keys, glasses, wallet, purse, phone, briefcase, and so on. What differentiates these from being normal, typical memory lapses versus a sign of a more serious problem is related to their frequency, severity, whether they interfere with life, and whether they represent a change. The same problem, say, spending an hour three times a week hunting for a pair of glasses, can be normal for someone who has hunted for things regularly all their lives. But for someone who never misplaced things more than once or twice a year, it would represent a significant change, signaling something abnormal.

REPEATING QUESTIONS AND STORIES MAY BE A SIGN OF RAPID FORGETTING

"You mentioned that there were a bunch of problems related to memory. What were some of the others?" Sue asks.

"Repeating herself," Sam sighs. "She started repeating questions, things she wanted to tell me, and stories at dinner parties. At first I thought it was the normal repetition that anyone can do by mistake. Take the dinner party stories. She would get a story in her mind, maybe something from high school about when she and her friend went to a dance and ended up two states away. It's a great story, but she might try to tell the same story to the same people two or three times. Or she would tell me what she learned at the hairdresser four times in an hour. Mind you, I wasn't really interested in hearing it once, so I would tell her, 'Mary, you've already told me that.' Then she might ask me who we were meeting for dinner, and I'd tell her, and then she would ask me again—and again—so I would tell her, 'Mary, you've asked me that same question three times in the last fifteen minutes.'"

Repeating questions and stories is often a sign of rapid forgetting, one of the hallmarks of Alzheimer's disease. Although anyone can forget they've said something, ask a question again, or forget the answer to a question, those with Alzheimer's disease tend to repeat things more frequently. They appear to have rapidly forgotten that they have already just told that story or asked that question. Another example of rapid forgetting is when something important is left unattended, such as the stove being left on or the water running. If these problems happen more often than previously, it is usually a sign of rapid forgetting.

ALZHEIMER'S DISEASE DAMAGES THE HIPPOCAMPUS

We'll discuss more about Alzheimer's disease in Step 3, Chapter 8, but for now the important thing to know is that it is the most common cause of rapid forgetting. Even as one gets older, rapid forgetting is not normal. If rapid forgetting is present, it should always be evaluated, as it may indicate Alzheimer's disease. Why does Alzheimer's cause rapid forgetting? Because Alzheimer's damages the hippocampus, where new memories are formed and stored. So in Alzheimer's, even if the frontal lobes are taking in new information related to episodes of our lives and sending it to the hippocampus, new memories are not forming (or are imperfectly forming) because the hippocampus is damaged.

DEPRESSION AND ANXIETY ARE COMMON WHEN ONE HAS MEMORY LOSS

"All that repetition must have been frustrating for you," Sue says sympathetically.

"I confess it was frustrating and annoying, but most of all it was very upsetting. She was so clearly having memory difficulties, and I didn't want to see it. I didn't want to admit to myself that she was having a problem. I also thought I could improve things by pointing out to her when she was repeating herself," Sam says, looking a bit upset himself now.

"Did it help, your telling her when she was repeating herself?"

"No. Unfortunately, I think correcting her just made her self-conscious about asking questions or saying anything. So she stopped wanting to go out to see other people for fear she would repeat herself. This was maybe two or three years ago. It was around this time that she started to get depressed."

There are few things that are as upsetting, depressing, and anxiety provoking as being aware that one has memory loss and worrying about Alzheimer's disease. We'll talk more about these issues in Steps 3 and 4, but for now we will just comment that depression and anxiety frequently result from individuals being aware of their memory loss.

NEW DIFFICULTIES WITH PLANNING AND ORGANIZING MAY SUGGEST A PROBLEM

"I did notice that Mary stopped giving her fabulous dinner parties," Sue says. "Did she stop hosting them because she was feeling depressed?"

"Actually, that happened earlier," Sam explains. "She simply wasn't able to do all of the planning and organizing needed to host a big dinner party. You might not have realized it, but the last one was quite difficult for her."

"Now that you mention it, I do recall that she was pretty stressed during that party, not relaxed and enjoying herself like usual."

Difficulty with planning and organizing events and activities, such as hosting dinner parties, making vacation plans, or hooking up new electronic devices, may be one of the earliest signs that something is wrong, whether the problem is due to Alzheimer's disease or another disorder. Such activities require many cognitive abilities—including memory—to be working together in a coordinated fashion.

DIFFICULTY FINDING ORDINARY WORDS CAN INDICATE A PROBLEM

"The other thing I noticed at that party was that Mary was quieter than usual. Was that because she was worried about repeating herself?" Sue asks.

"No," Sam replies. "At that time it was more trouble finding words that made her feel a bit uncomfortable talking. And I don't mean just people's names. She was having trouble finding ordinary words like . . ." Sam looks around the table, "cup, spoon, sugar . . . stuff like that. She found it embarrassing when she couldn't come up with a word, and she didn't like it when people filled in the word for her."

Word-finding difficulties are extremely common in Alzheimer's disease. Whereas in normal aging there is difficulty coming up with names of people, places, books, movies, and other proper nouns, in Alzheimer's there is difficulty coming up with ordinary, common nouns of everyday things. These difficulties may manifest as the wrong or less precise term being used (e.g., shoe for sandal, bread for bagel) or, more commonly, simply as pauses in sentences when the word is searched for. Friends and families often get used to jumping in during these pauses to provide the missing word.

Sue thinks about everything that Sam had just told her about Mary's early symptoms. *Did she herself have any of these problems? She certainly got lost sometimes, but she was usually able to find her way back without too much difficulty. She did often misplace her glasses and her datebook. Was she misplacing them more than before? She's not sure. She knows she isn't entertaining the way she used to. Is that a sign of the start of Alzheimer's disease? She has also noticed trouble coming up with people's names—much more than she used to. Sue can understand why Mary became depressed. Worrying about Alzheimer's is enough to make anyone depressed.*

"So those were the main problems that Mary had when it started," continues Sam, interrupting Sue's thoughts. "Anything else you want to know?"

"Thanks, Sam, no, that was very helpful," Sue replies, turning her attention back to him. "It's always hard to know what memory problems are normal, being our age, and which could be signs of Alzheimer's. Now I have a much better sense."

"Anytime. I mean that. Just let me know if you have any more questions. And my advice to you is that if you have any concerns about your memory, get it checked out. Don't let your doctor put you off if you are concerned you might have a problem."

"Thanks again, Sam, I really appreciate your advice."

SUMMARY

In this chapter we learned about the thinking and memory problems that are common in Alzheimer's disease, including getting lost, losing things, trouble with planning and organizing, and difficulties finding words. We learned that whereas normal aging damages the frontal lobes, leading to difficulties in learning and retrieving information, Alzheimer's disease damages the hippocampus, leading to rapid forgetting: information—even when learned—is lost permanently within days, hours, or even minutes. We also learned that depression and anxiety are common in Alzheimer's disease.

Let's now review some of the memory issues raised in the Introduction as well as others that could be caused by Alzheimer's disease.

- A week after seeing a movie you have trouble remembering the name of the movie and parts of the plot.
  - We discussed in the last chapter that having difficulty recalling the name of a movie may simply be related to normal aging. Not remembering major parts of the plot, however, could be a sign of rapid forgetting (assuming that you were paying attention to the movie as you were watching it), which could, in turn, indicate Alzheimer's disease.
- You spend too much time looking for your keys, glasses, wallet, or purse.

- o If you are now spending much more time hunting down items compared to how much time you spent in the past—particularly if is interfering with your being on time for activities—it could be an early sign of Alzheimer's disease.
- Your family tells you that you've asked that question before.
  - o Repeating questions may be due to rapid forgetting, which could be a sign of Alzheimer's disease.
- You're driving a route you have done more than twenty times before, but this time you become lost and cannot get to where you want to go without calling someone for help.
  - o Getting lost and having great difficulty getting straightened out and back on track is always concerning if it is a route that you have done many times before, even if you haven't driven that route for a while.
- You've done household repairs all of your life, and even put in a whole bathroom, including plumbing and electrical work. Although you can still change a light bulb, you now find you cannot fix much else around the house.
  - o No longer being able to do common activities that you have done all your life because of problems with thinking or memory is always a concern.
- Although you've never been good with people's names, you now find yourself having such difficulties finding common words that other people are filling them in and finishing your sentences.
  - o Word-finding difficulties prominent enough to cause others to jump in and help you out with ordinary words—not just names—is concerning.
- You've been worried about your memory loss and have begun to feel depressed and anxious about it. Your spouse encourages you to get it checked out, but your best friend thinks it's not any worse than his and suggests you ignore it.
  - o If you are worried about your memory enough that you are becoming anxious or depressed, get it checked out.

By now you should have a sense as to which of your memory problems are likely due to normal aging and which, if any, could be concerning for Alzheimer's disease. In Chapter 4 we'll learn more about the patterns of memory loss seen in normal aging versus Alzheimer's and the basics of what your doctor can do to evaluate your memory problems.

4

What Should the Doctor Do to Evaluate My Memory?

In this chapter we'll learn more about the patterns of memory loss that everyone experiences as they grow older versus those brought on by Alzheimer's disease. We'll also review some basic steps your doctor should take to evaluate your memory.

MEMORY PROBLEMS THAT AFFECT YOUR ACTIVITIES OR FUNCTION SHOULD ALWAYS BE EVALUATED

When we last saw Jack, he was telling his daughter, Sara, that he was concerned about his memory and had just decided to get it checked out. Let's catch up with Jack now as he visits his regular doctor.

Jack fidgets uncomfortably in the exam room. *I'm nervous,* he thinks to himself. That surprises him. He likes his doctor and rarely feels uncomfortable seeing her. *I guess this memory loss and Alzheimer's stuff has gotten to me*, he concludes, frowning.

After a few more minutes of fidgeting, his doctor comes in.

"Hi, Jack, nice to see you. What brings you in to see me today?" the doctor asks.

"I'm worried about my memory, Doc," Jack replies.

"Oh, what problems have you noticed with your memory?"

"It isn't that bad, but I'm definitely having more trouble than I used to when I try to remember things."

"Can you recall any specific examples of when your memory let you down?"

"Yes," Jack replies, "I was just mentioning some things to my daughter. I think I've always had a good memory. I've spent nearly my whole life as an electrician going to different people's houses and never had any difficulty remembering an address, but now I need to go over a new address about ten times before I can learn it. The same thing happens if I'm trying to remember an appointment . . . I need to go over it a bunch of times before I can remember it."

"Any other problems?" she asks, not sounding too concerned.

"Yeah, I've got a lot of trouble coming up with names—even names of my buddies that I've known for years."

"Trouble recalling people's names is quite common as one gets older, and isn't usually associated with a disorder," she says reassuringly. "Anything else you've noticed?"

"The other thing that is happening is that I keep showing up in the wrong place or at the wrong time for something. Just last week I went to the lodge to meet Sam for lunch, but it turns out I was supposed to meet him at the diner. It was only when he called me on my cell phone that we sorted it out."

"So you went to the wrong place for your lunch date?" she says, suddenly sounding concerned. "Have there been other times that you have made that type of error and missed or been late for an appointment?"

"Well, I'm not sure if I've missed any, but I did show up on the wrong day to pick up my granddaughter from soccer practice. I'm there on Monday afternoon in the middle school fields looking for her and all I see are boys. I ask someone where the girls are playing, and she tells me that the girls play on Tuesday. When I got home, I looked at the calendar and saw that I was supposed to pick her up on Tuesday, not Monday. So I went back the next day," Jack explains.

"OK, Jack. Thanks for going through those examples with me. Everything you have told me could be related to the normal changes that occur in the brain when one gets older. But the fact that your memory difficulties have impacted some of your activities—meeting your friend for lunch, picking up your granddaughter—makes me think we should check it out."

As we discussed in Step 1, Chapter 2, there are some types of memory problems that may simply be due to normal aging but that could also signal more serious problems. One rule of thumb when deciding whether a memory problem should be evaluated is if memory problems are interfering with your activities. If you find that you are missing appointments or showing up in the wrong place or at the wrong time for appointments, you should have your memory evaluated. As we will discuss in the remaining five Steps, once we understand what the problem is with your memory, we will be able to help you learn what you can do to improve your memory and your day-to-day functioning. An evaluation by your doctor may be important to help you understand whether anything is wrong with your memory and, if so, the different treatment options available. More on these topics later—read on!

OLDER MEMORIES ARE STORED IN THE CORTEX OF THE BRAIN

"I'm actually glad to hear you say that, Doc. I want to get my memory sorted out so I can stop worrying about it. I've got this buddy, Sam, down at the lodge whose wife has Alzheimer's, and he told me he is worried that I might be developing Alzheimer's, too. You don't think it's Alzheimer's, do you, Doc? I mean, I could tell you what cars each of my friends drove in high school. You can't have Alzheimer's and remember things from so long ago, can you?" Jack asks nervously.

"Let's not get ahead of ourselves," the doctor says evenly. "We need to do the workup and see what it shows. But to answer your question, Alzheimer's disease mainly affects the formation of new memories, leaving the older memories intact. I want to be clear—I'm not saying that I think you have Alzheimer's disease—but individuals with Alzheimer's can often remember everything from high school quite well, just not what happened yesterday or last week."

In the prior chapters we introduced two parts of the brain related to memory: the frontal lobes that pay attention, organize, and help to facilitate storage and retrieval of memories, and the hippocampus that binds and temporarily stores new memories. Now we will introduce the last component, the cortex, the outer layer of the brain. When a new memory is formed—let's say your memory for the dinner you had last night—the frontal lobes, by paying attention to the dinner, facilitate the binding and temporary storage of the memory in the hippocampus. This memory of your dinner will be bound and stored in the hippocampus for a few days or weeks (or sometimes longer) until it slowly gets transformed into a more permanent memory with the other older memories in the cortex, a process known as "consolidation." We don't know a lot about consolidation, but we do know that it requires several stages of sleep (including rapid-eye-movement or REM sleep), which is one of the reasons that good sleep is important for memory function (for more on sleep, see Step 5, Chapter 13).

OLDER MEMORIES IN THE CORTEX ARE RELATIVELY UNAFFECTED IN EARLY ALZHEIMER'S DISEASE

In the last chapter we discussed how Alzheimer's disease affects the hippocampus, leading to rapid forgetting. Older memories in the cortex, however, are relatively spared by Alzheimer's, particularly early on. Thus, the classic pattern of memory loss in early Alzheimer's disease is impairment in the binding and storage of new memories in the hippo-campus, rapid forgetting of recently formed memories in the hippocampus, and preservation of the older memories in the cortex.

BLOOD WORK AND BRAIN IMAGING ARE KEY TOOLS FOR EVALUATING POSSIBLE CAUSES OF MEMORY LOSS

"OK, I get it," Jack says, crestfallen. "Just because I can remember things from high school doesn't mean I don't have Alzheimer's." With more resolve in his voice he continues, "So how can we sort it out? What do I need to do? Do you need to take a piece of my brain? I read somewhere that is the only way to know for sure . . . I'm ready, Doc."

"No, we're not going to take a piece of your brain," she replies, smiling, "although I don't deny that would settle the issue of whether you had Alzheimer's disease. I thought we would start by getting a picture of your brain—an MRI or a cat scan—and drawing some blood."

"Can you see the Alzheimer's on the scan or in the blood?"

"No, you can't be sure that someone has Alzheimer's disease just by looking at an MRI or CT scan or doing blood work, but you can rule out other possible causes of memory loss."

Alzheimer's disease is not the only disorder that erodes memory. Many other types of problems can also cause memory loss, so it is important for your doctor to look for signs of abnormalities in your blood and in your brain. The laboratory studies of your blood should include basic tests to make sure there are no signs of infections or problems in your blood chemistry, in addition to some special tests to make sure there are no vitamin deficiencies or problems with your thyroid. Two basic brain imaging scans can get a good picture of the structure of your brain: magnetic resonance imaging (MRI) and computed tomography (CT or "cat" scans). MRIs use a powerful magnet to look at the brain. MRIs give better pictures than CT scans, which use X-rays, but either test will show whether there is anything wrong with the structure of the brain. We'll go over the specific problems that you can find in the blood work and brain imaging scans in more detail in Step 3, Chapter 6.

QUESTIONNAIRES CAN BE HELPFUL IN CHARACTERIZING AND SCREENING FOR MEMORY PROBLEMS

"I'll also have you sit down with my nurse to do a little paper-and-pencil test of your thinking and memory. We can do the test today if you have a few extra minutes," the doctor continues.

"A test!" Jack responds with alarm, "I thought there might be a test. If I don't pass it, does that mean I have Alzheimer's? I'm no good at tests, Doc, never was."

"No, it won't mean that you have Alzheimer's disease in particular, just that something isn't right with your thinking and memory. Do your best, and we'll go over the results when I see you back in three to four weeks."

After fifteen minutes in the waiting room, the nurse brings Jack into an exam room and explains, "First, I'm going to ask you some questions about whether you have noticed any changes in the last several years caused by thinking and memory problems."

"OK, shoot," Jack responds.

"*Have you noticed any problems with judgment?* For example, any problems making decisions, bad financial decisions, or problems with thinking?"

"No, I don't think so. I get my pension from the union each month and my house is paid off, so I don't have a lot of financial decisions to make," Jack responds.

"OK, got it. *Have you had less interest in hobbies or activities?*"

"Well, that's a tough one . . . I was working up until about three or four years ago, and I never really had any hobbies. But I mow the grass and do chores around the house like always, and still go play hockey with the guys."

"OK, we'll say 'no' to that one, too. *Do you find you repeat the same things over and over, such as questions, stories, or statements?*"

"No, I don't think so . . . at least, no one told me that I do."

"*What about any trouble learning how to use a tool, appliance, or gadget, such as a VCR, computer, microwave, or remote control?*"

"Well, I can use any tool you could throw at me, but a computer—forget it! They tried to teach me computers the last year I was in my job, and I just couldn't get the hang of it. That was one of the reasons I retired. Stupid computers."

"Computers certainly can be frustrating," she agrees, checking "yes" on her sheet. "*Do you ever forget what month or year it is?*"

"Month or year? No. I might be off on the date, but not month or year."

"*Do you have any trouble handling complicated financial affairs, such as balancing your checkbook, doing your income taxes, or paying bills?*"

"No, I don't think I've ever been late paying a bill, and my checkbook is always balanced. My daughter has been helping me with the taxes ever since my wife died."

"OK, good. *Do you have any trouble remembering appointments?*" she asks.

"You've got me on that one," Jack responds. "I was telling the
doctor that I'm having a lot of trouble remembering appointments. Lately I've been showing up in the wrong place or at
the wrong time."

"OK, got it," she says, checking another "yes" on her sheet.
"Last question: *Do you have daily problems with thinking and/
or memory?*"

"Daily problems? No, I don't think I have daily problems with
thinking or memory."

"OK, Jack, that's great. We've finished the first thing we have
to do."

Questionnaires about day-to-day functioning help characterize
the nature of memory problems, as well as screening for memory disorders. The AD8 is an eight-item questionnaire designed
to detect problems that could be related to changes in thinking
and memory caused by Alzheimer's disease or another cause of
memory loss. The eight questions are italicized in the preceding dialogue and listed at the end of the chapter. The doctors
who developed the test found that most people who responded
"yes" to none or just one of the questions were aging normally,
whereas most people who responded "yes" to two or more questions had some type of brain disorder, such as Alzheimer's disease. The AD8 is one of a number of excellent questionnaires
available that can be completed by an individual with concerns
about memory or, more commonly, by a family member. See
Further Reading for additional details.

COGNITIVE TESTING IS ESSENTIAL IN THE EVALUATION OF MEMORY PROBLEMS

Jack relaxes for a minute after finishing the questionnaire as the
nurse pulls out some papers. She folds one of the sheets of

paper so that Jack can see the top half of it. On the paper Jack can see some dots with numbers and letters inside them and line drawings of a shape and some animals.

"What's this?" Jack asks.

"It's a brief test of your thinking and memory." Then, seeing the anxiety on Jack's face, she adds, "Not to worry, just do your best. By the way, how far through school did you go?"

"All the way," Jack states. When she doesn't respond he adds, "twelfth grade." "Great, thanks," she says, writing twelve at the top of the page. She then pulls out another sheet of paper and reads: "The first thing I'd like you to do is to draw a line going from a number to a letter in ascending order. Begin here, and draw a line from 1 then to A then to 2 and so on. End here."

Oh, I get it, Jack says to himself, *we need to alternate numbers and letters.*

Jack does this alternating connect-the-dots test, and then other things that the nurse asks him to do, including copying the shape, drawing a clock, and naming the animals. She then takes the piece of paper away and asks him to remember five words, going over the words with him twice. He's pleased that he could repeat all five of the words back to her. She sets a timer and informs him she will ask about the words again at the end of the test. Next she asks him to repeat numbers forwards and backwards, to tap with his hand when he hears a certain letter, and to count backwards from eighty by sevens. She then has him repeat some sentences and say all the words he can think of that begin with the letter B. She asks him how several pairs of different things are alike.

Jack finds he has a bit of trouble with a couple of the tasks. Somehow his brain didn't want to do things backwards, whether it was repeating numbers backwards or counting backwards by sevens. Then the timer goes off and she asks him to recall those five words. He thinks and thinks, trying to remember. "I'm sorry but I cannot recall any of them," Jack says, clearly upset with himself.

"Not to worry," she responds. She then adds as if they were sharing a secret, "I'll give you some hints. One of them was something you eat."

"Egg!" Jack exclaims.

"Right!" she responds, encouragingly.

She continues to give Jack hints, and he is pleased that he is able to get another word with this type of hint, and one more word when she gives him a list of three words to choose from.

"So I still missed two words," Jack says, clearly disappointed with himself.

"That's OK," she says kindly. "The doctor asked me to give you these tests because you told her you were having trouble with your memory. If you did perfectly on the tests, it would mean that they are not sensitive enough to detect your problem. The fact that you had trouble on some of the items means that we are giving you the right tests. Speaking of the test, I've got just a few more questions to ask you. What's today's date?"

Jack gives her the date, and then she asks the month, year, day of the week, place they are in, and their city. Jack is off by one on the date.

"How'd I do?" Jack asks nervously.

"You did fine," she says reassuringly. "You missed one point for saying the numbers in backwards order, one for doing those subtractions by seven, five for the words, and one for the date . . ."

"But I only missed two of the words!" Jack interjects.

"Yes, but that was after I gave you some hints. We still score it by whether you could recall the words without hints."

"Oh," Jack says, disappointed again.

"You got 22 points, but we give you an extra point for your education, so you scored 23 out of 30."

"I get an extra point for graduating high school?"

"Actually, you get an extra point for not doing more education than high school."

"First time I was ever rewarded for not going to college!" Jack responds, laughing. He continues, more soberly, "So is 23 OK? Or does it mean I have Alzheimer's?"

"Well, it's just a bit below the cutoff of 26. So it does suggest that your thinking and memory are not doing as well as when you were younger."

Tests that evaluate thinking and memory are key to identifying memory problems that are due to more than just normal aging. Different patterns of performance can suggest different disorders, allowing doctors to characterize and identify the memory problem. Some of these tests can also be used to screen for memory disorders in individuals without particular memory complaints.

MEMORY DISORDERS SUCH AS ALZHEIMER'S DISEASE ARE VERY COMMON AS WE AGE

Jack thinks about the nurse's words, "... *your thinking and memory are not doing as well as when you were younger."*

He then says out loud, a bit defensively, "Well, I know my memory isn't as good as when I was younger, but is it really abnormal? I bet half the people I know have similar difficulties."

"Well, I'm not an expert," the nurse replies, "but my understanding is that as they get older many people develop memory disorders and most of them don't even know it. So you might be right that many people you know have memory problems—probably many of them should also get their memory checked out."

Jack doesn't respond right away. He is thinking to himself, *I would be one of those people with memory problems and not know it, if Sam hadn't said something to me . . .*

Just as heart disease, cancer, and diabetes occur more frequently as we get older, memory problems due to Alzheimer's disease and other disorders also become more common with age. It is estimated that approximately half of people aged eighty-five years or older have Alzheimer's or another disorder causing memory loss. Just because a friend's memory is as bad as ours doesn't mean that our memory problems should be ignored.

SUMMARY

Memory disorders become more common as we get older. If your memory problems are interfering with your activities or your function, you should definitely have your memory evaluated. Older memories are stored in the cortex, and these older memories remain intact and available in early Alzheimer's disease. The basic parts of an evaluation for memory disorders include blood work, an MRI or CT scan, questionnaires, and cognitive testing.

Let's now consider some examples to illustrate what we learned in this chapter.

- You've been worrying about your memory problems for more than a year. In the last couple of months, there have been a few slips: one where you forgot about a lunch date with your friend, and another where you got turned around trying to get to a store, got lost, and ended up driving back home. You're wondering if it is time to get your memory evaluated.
  - Yes! If your memory problems are interfering with day-to-day aspects of your life, you should definitely have them evaluated.
- You just had another "senior moment" where you forgot what you were supposed to be doing. You've also noted some difficulties coming up with words, and you are spending more time hunting through your house looking for things you've lost. However, most of your friends are having the same problems, so it must just be normal aging, right?
  - Not necessarily. Memory disorders such as Alzheimer's disease are common as we get older. If you are having significant problems and your friend is, too, it may be that you both should have your memories checked out.
- You are having some difficulties remembering recent events, such as who you went to the movies with last week and where you went

to dinner before the show. However, you can still remember many things from your childhood and teenage years such as the house you grew up in, your high school teachers, and some of the dances you used to go to with your friends. If your memory is good enough to remember things from high school, it must not be Alzheimer's, right?

- o Actually, the typical pattern of memory loss due to Alzheimer's disease is that the older memories are relatively preserved; it is the recent memories that are impaired. Remembering your childhood well but having difficulties remembering what happened last week would be consistent with a disorder such as Alzheimer's disease.

• You've mentioned your memory issues to your doctor, and he wants to get an MRI scan and blood work. However, you're claustrophobic and hate needles. Should you tell your doctor that you don't want these parts of the evaluation?

- o No! The brain imaging study and blood work are important parts of the evaluation for memory problems. Most people do just fine in the MRI scanner by simply closing their eyes and relaxing. There are also "open MRI" scanners that have a larger tube. You can always have a CT scan instead; CT scanners are very open and the scans are quick (usually under five minutes).

• Your doctor wants you to take a test of your thinking and memory. However, you don't want to take the test, and, in any event, you get test anxiety, so the test results will probably not be valid. Should you take the test anyways?

- o Yes. Tests of thinking and memory are an important part of the evaluation of memory loss. The pattern of performance due to anxiety on a memory test is different from that due to a memory disorder, so the test results will still be helpful even if you are anxious.

• You would like to screen yourself for memory problems before you bring a memory issue up with anyone else, even your doctor. Can you actually screen yourself for memory problems?

- o Yes. Many questionnaires can be used as self-screening tools. You just need to be sure that you can be honest with yourself. Want to see how you would do on the AD8, the questionnaire we referred to in this chapter? Simply ask yourself the following questions. If you answer "yes, this is a change" to two or more of these items, we recommend that you make an appointment to see your doctor to discuss your memory problems.

AD8 Dementia Screening Interview*

1. Problems with judgment (e.g., problems making decisions, bad financial decisions, problems with thinking)
2. Less interest in hobbies/activities
3. Repeats the same things over and over (questions, stories, or statements)
4. Trouble learning how to use a tool, appliance, or gadget (e.g., VCR, computer, microwave, remote control)
5. Forgets correct month or year
6. Trouble handling complicated financial affairs (e.g., balancing checkbook, income taxes, paying bills)
7. Trouble remembering appointments
8. Daily problems with thinking and/or memory

Now that we have covered the components of a basic memory evaluation as carried out by a primary care provider, we are ready to turn to Chapter 5 to understand when a more specialized evaluation is necessary and what that special evaluation consists of.

* Adapted from J. E. Galvin et al. (2005). The AD8, a brief informant interview to detect dementia. *Neurology, 65,* 559–564. Copyright 2005. The AD8 is a copyrighted instrument of the Alzheimer's Disease Research Center, Washington University, St. Louis, Missouri. All Rights Reserved.

5

When Are Special Tests and Evaluations Needed?

Most evaluations of thinking and memory can be performed by your primary care provider. Sometimes, however, evaluations by specialists are needed. In this chapter and the next we'll discuss when these specialist evaluations are needed and how they typically work.

IF YOU ARE CONCERNED ABOUT YOUR MEMORY, GET IT CHECKED OUT

When we last saw Sue she was meeting with Sam to learn more about some of the problems that his wife, Mary, had when she started to show signs of Alzheimer's disease. After hearing about Mary's problems with thinking and memory, Sue worries that some of her own problems are similar, and so she is taking Sam's advice to see her doctor. Let's check in on Sue now as she gets ready to see her physician.

Sue looks at her date book. First she will see her doctor at 9:15. Then she has her beauty shop appointment at 11:00. She will meet her friends for lunch at the mall at 12:30. *If the doctor is on time and I don't make any wrong turns, the timing should work out fine*, she thinks to herself. Just to be sure, she goes to her computer and prints out a map with the locations of each of her appointments. *Yes, even with a bit of traffic everything should work.* She decides to slip the map along with her appointment book into her purse. Just in case. Then she opens her address book and looks at the notes she had written about her friends, to remind herself of important information that might come up when she meets with them—such as the names of their spouses and children and what they do. She slips her address book into her purse as well.

She drives to her doctor's office without needing to consult the map.

"Thanks so much for seeing me before my regular checkup," Sue says to her physician. She then adds tentatively, "I don't know if something is wrong, but I've become increasingly concerned about my memory."

"What problems have you noticed?" her doctor asks.

"Everything is just more difficult than it used to be, even compared to just a couple of years ago. I'm still able to do my shopping, pay my bills, and balance my checkbook. It's just that all these activities take longer than they used to, and seem to need more effort," Sue explains. "Is that normal for someone my age?"

"It certainly could be," he responds. "Have you experienced any other difficulties? Any trouble with appointments?"

"It's the same thing. I haven't missed any that I know of, but I need to spend much more time keeping track of and preparing for appointments than I used to. I'm pretty sure that I would have missed some if I weren't being extra careful."

In Chapter 4 we mentioned that memory problems that affect your activities or function should always be evaluated. But that isn't the only reason to have your memory checked out. Another reason to get an evaluation is when you or someone you know well is concerned about your memory. Don't wait until memory problems progress enough to impair your function before you seek an evaluation.

NEEDING MORE EFFORT TO PERFORM ACTIVITIES CAN BE AN EARLY SIGN OF MEMORY LOSS

Are you finding that it is more difficult for you to carry out the activities that make up your weekly routine? There are many reasons why routine activities that depend upon thinking and memory may be more difficult for you now than they used to be. As we discussed, in normal aging our older frontal lobes are simply not as efficient as they used to be. So it can be perfectly normal to have more difficulties doing routine tasks as we get older.

It is also true, however, that when viewed from hindsight, most individuals with established memory disorders who are currently unable to do one or more daily activities went through an intermediate stage when they were still able to do the activities if they put in more effort. So it is important to notice when greater effort is required to do our usual activities. How do we know when the need for greater effort is part of normal aging or whether it may be a sign of a memory disorder? It can be tricky, and often the specialists discussed in this chapter and the next are needed to answer that question.

SCREENING TESTS MAY NOT BE ACCURATE FOR SOMEONE WHO IS HIGHLY EDUCATED, IS VERY BRIGHT, HAS A LEARNING DISABILITY, OR HAS A DIFFERENT CULTURAL BACKGROUND

"How's your memory doing?" asks the doctor.

"Well, on the one hand, I feel it is terrible. I cannot recall things like I used to be able to when I was younger. And when it comes to names, forget it—I have trouble remembering the names of people I've known for years. But on the other hand, I know a lot of my friends are experiencing similar things, so then I think maybe that's normal," Sue answers.

"Remind me, Sue, you went to college, correct?"

"Yes, and then I received a master's degree in education after that."

"OK, here's what I think we should do. I've learned a few things about memory disorders over the last couple of years. You're a very bright woman. Although I could give you some brief tests of thinking and memory here in the office, I worry that they may not be sensitive enough to pick up any subtle deficits that you may have. In other words, because you're quite smart, you could score in the normal range on these tests and still be having some small but real problems. Because I don't want to miss any potentially treatable disorders, I'm going to refer you to a specialized memory center where I know the neurologists and neuropsychologists can carefully evaluate your thinking and memory."

Because we need to take intelligence as well as other factors such as someone's culture, occupation, and any prior learning disabilities into account when interpreting tests of thinking and memory, screening tests that can be performed quickly in a primary care setting are not the right test for everyone. Sometimes the screening test will suggest that a memory disorder is present when in actuality the problem is a lifelong learning disability or another factor. Screening tests also often miss small but very real signs of memory loss in someone with particularly high baseline thinking and memory function. In these cases it is best to see a neuropsychologist or other memory specialist.

NEUROPSYCHOLOGISTS EVALUATE THINKING, MEMORY, AND BEHAVIOR

A few weeks have passed and Sue and her husband, John, are sitting in the waiting room of the memory center. "I'm not exactly sure why they wanted you to come with me, but

I'm glad to have you here," Sue says to John as she takes his hand in hers.

"And I'm glad to be here with you," John answers as he squeezes her hand gently.

A few minutes later, one of the doctors introduces herself to Sue and John and brings them back to her office. "Please have a seat," she says in a friendly manner, gesturing to two chairs as they walk into the room. "It's nice to meet you both. I'm a neuropsychologist. That means I specialize in understanding how brain diseases can impact thinking, memory, and behavior, by talking to you both and through pencil-and-paper tests and questionnaires."

Sue nods, a bit nervously.

The neuropsychologist continues, "The way that we typically begin our evaluations here at the memory center is by talking to you," she says as she looks at Sue, "so that I can get a good understanding of all the different problems that you have noticed with your thinking and memory. I'll also ask you some more general questions to get to know your background better. Then I'll have you work with one of my assistants who will spend about one and a half to two hours with you doing some pencil-and-paper tests of your thinking and memory. When we score the tests, we will compare your results to those of people the same age with a similar background to see if you are performing how we would expect. While you are doing those tests, if it is OK with you, I'd like to spend a few minutes chatting with your husband about what changes he has observed in your thinking and memory. That will be enough for one day. But before you go, we will set you up for an MRI scan of your brain and some blood work. When you come back, you will first meet with our neurologist for a medical and neurological evaluation and to go over your MRI and blood work. Then you'll meet back with me again to review the pencil-and-paper test results, sum up our thoughts of your evaluation, and— most importantly—discuss what we can do to help. How does that sound for a plan?"

"Sounds great," Sue says out loud as she thinks to herself, *Finally I'm going to understand if there is something wrong with my memory or not.*

Neuropsychologists are psychologists who have received advanced training in the use and interpretation of pencil-and-paper tests and questionnaires to help diagnose brain disorders. Neuropsychological evaluations factor in how many or few years of education someone has, cultural differences, any prior learning disabilities, any current or prior psychiatric disorders, and other factors that could impact an individual's ability to perform well on tests of thinking and memory. For most tests, instead of a simple "passing" or "failing" score, results are compared to those of other people who are the same age and have a similar background. So the same test result could be normal for an eighty-year-old but could represent a problem for someone age fifty. Once they better understand the relative strengths and weaknesses of someone's thinking and memory, neuropsychologists also make specific recommendations of things that people can do to improve their function in daily life.

THE INTERVIEW SEEKS PROBLEMS THAT COULD BE CONCERNING FOR ALZHEIMER'S OR ANOTHER DISEASE

"So what difficulties are you having with your thinking and memory that led your physician to refer you to us?"

Sue begins by explaining the same issues that she mentioned to her doctor: how daily activities are more difficult and take more effort than before, how her memory doesn't seem as good as when she was younger, and how she has great difficulties coming up with people's names quickly to the point that it is sometimes embarrassing.

"Are there any other problems you've noticed with your memory? Have you ever left the stove on? Do you find yourself asking the same questions or telling the same stories again?"

"No, I don't think I'm doing any of those things," responds Sue, looking over to her husband, John, for confirmation.

"No, I haven't seen any of those problems," John agrees.

"Have you noticed any problems finding your words—not just names but common, ordinary words like 'desk' and 'chair'?" continues the neuropsychologist as she gestures to the furniture in the room.

Sue thinks. "No, I don't think I'm having trouble with ordinary words . . . at least not any more trouble than I have had for the last thirty years or so," she responds.

"How about any trouble getting lost?"

"No, but I do take a look at where I am going on a map before I head out, particularly if it's someplace new or if I haven't been there in a while."

"Any trouble planning and organizing activities?"

"Well, that's another thing that takes a lot more effort than it used to. I don't have difficulty planning a dinner for a few friends, but I confess I don't have the energy to plan big parties or charity events like I did in the past."

"OK, so no trouble planning and organizing small parties, but perhaps some difficulty in organizing large functions?"

"Yes, that sounds right," Sue confirms. "It now feels overwhelming to plan a large event."

"Have you noticed any changes in your mood?"

"Not really . . . other than being anxious about my memory," Sue confesses.

"Well, that's completely understandable. Hopefully by the time we've finished with our evaluation, you will understand what's going on with your memory so you won't need to feel anxious about it."

Changing tone slightly, the neuropsychologist continues: "OK, so the main problems are that you feel your memory isn't as good as when you were younger, you have difficulty coming up with people's names, it takes more effort to do your usual activities, and it now feels overwhelming to plan and organize large events. You also feel somewhat anxious about your memory. Does that sound right?"

"Yes, that's a good summary," Sue confirms.

"OK, now I'm going to ask you a few background questions. You're eighty years old, correct?"

Sue nods.

"How far did you go through school?"

"I have a master's degree in education."

"That's wonderful. Did you teach?"

"I taught eighth-grade English for about ten years, before our children were born."

"I bet that was challenging!"

"I enjoyed that age—the students are exploring who they are," Sue explains.

"Did you work outside the home after that?"

"Not for money, but I did some work at local charities, and I used to organize fundraising events."

"Great, that's helpful. Now come with me and I'll introduce you to my assistant, who will work with you on the pencil-and-paper tests we spoke about." Turning to John, the neuropsychologist says, "Please wait in my office for a minute. I'll be right back, and we can chat a little about your impressions of how your wife's thinking and memory are doing."

After beginning with a more general question, neuropsychologists and other memory specialists will ask about specific thinking and memory problems that may suggest a brain disorder. These basic questions will include asking about the same thinking and memory problems that we learned are signs of Alzheimer's disease in Step 2, Chapter 3.

BRING FAMILY (OR A CLOSE FRIEND) TO THE EVALUATION

After a minute the neuropsychologist returns to the office and asks John, "So, what are your impressions of how your wife is doing in regards to her thinking and memory?"

"I think she's doing pretty well for eighty years old," John replies. "I mean, everybody our age has some memory problems, right?"

"Let me ask you a slightly different question. Do you think her ability to remember has declined over the last several years?"

"Well, you need to know that Sue is very bright, and she has always had an amazing memory. She's very modest, so she wouldn't tell you, but I think she got straight A's in college. And those charity events she mentioned—those were very big events that coordinated several organizations. What I can tell you is that her memory used to be much better than mine. She would be able to remember her grocery and shopping lists in her head. Not me—I have always had to write everything down. For the last couple of years I have noticed that she also needs to write things down on lists or she may not remember it. Mind you, she doesn't have trouble with the shopping, but I do think it is a change that she now depends upon lists," John responds.

"That's very helpful. Are there any other changes you've noticed?"

"The only other thing I have noticed is that she is not as quick to pick up on new technology, whether it is a new website she is trying to navigate or a new phone she has bought—although I confess I've always been the tech-savvy one in our home."

"Have you noticed any changes in her behavior or personality?"

"No, nothing like that. She's the same Sue."

"How do you feel her mood is? Do you think she could be depressed?"

"Well, that's a good question. She is really nervous about her memory, like she said. She might be depressed; I'm not sure. She doesn't have a lot of energy these days, but who does at age eighty!"

"OK, thanks for this information. The last thing I'd like you to do is to fill out this questionnaire regarding her function. It includes questions about all sorts of activities of daily living, everything from eating and dressing to managing finances."

"Will do. Thanks for your help." John responds, shaking her hand and then taking the clipboard with the questionnaire on it.

"It is my pleasure. I'll see you back in two to three weeks after Sue has had her MRI, blood work, and she meets with the neurologist."

There are two main reasons that it is important for the doctor to speak with a family member or close friend when evaluating a memory problem. The first is that it is simply difficult when one has memory problems—even mild memory problems—to remember all of the times that things are forgotten. So you will want to bring someone with you who knows you well when you are going to have your memory evaluated.

The second reason is that speaking with a family member or friend might help identify changes in behavior or personality that the individual may not volunteer or even be aware of. These could include changes in diet, hygiene, or clothing. They might also include inappropriate, irritable, or aggressive behavior. These types of changes are very important for the doctor to know about, as they could indicate an unusual type of memory disorder that we will discuss later in Step 3, Chapter 10. Changes in behavior may also be important to know about so that they can be treated sooner rather than later.

NEUROPSYCHOLOGICAL TESTS EVALUATE ASPECTS OF THINKING AND MEMORY RELATED TO DIFFERENT BRAIN NETWORKS AND REGIONS

While the neuropsychologist was talking with John, Sue was getting started on the pencil-and-paper tests with her assistant.

"We're going to spend the next hour and a half or so going through some tests of your thinking and memory," the assistant explains. "One important thing to understand is that for most of the tests we are going to do, no one scores perfectly, so just because you make an error or have trouble with some parts, that doesn't mean that you are impaired or that there is anything wrong."

"You mean it is graded on a curve?" Sue asks.

"Yes, exactly. Your scores will be compared with those of other people who are about your age and who have roughly the same number of years of education."

"Well, that's reassuring," Sue says.

"Are you ready for the first test?"

"Sure, let's go."

"OK, so in this first test I'd simply like you to read each of these words out loud."

As Sue begins to read the words, she is aware that it is only because she is familiar with words like "knife" that she knows how to pronounce them correctly. Next Sue repeats some numbers in forward and backward order. Then she writes down abstract symbols corresponding to numbers in little boxes as fast as she can, using a code at the top of the page. She is then given two brief stories to remember and retell as accurately as she can right away, and then again about thirty minutes later, followed by learning a list of words to remember. In the next test she is given some lines, shapes, and figures to copy; some of the figures are simple and some are very complex. She is then asked to say as many words as she can think of that begin with the letter "W" in one minute, and then to say words that can begin with any letter but have to be in a specific category such as "colors." After that she is asked to name a series of line drawings. Next she does a few different connect-the-dots tests that become progressively more interesting.

Then she is asked to sort a special deck of cards. "But you haven't told me how to sort them," Sue notes.

"That's part of the test, for you to figure it out."

Lastly, she is given some questionnaires. Sue can see right away that these questionnaires are getting at whether she is feeling anxious or depressed. She answers them honestly.

Sue finds many of the tests interesting, although some are frustrating, and in others she feels rushed. "It's been a long time since I've taken a test. I'm glad you warned me that no one scores perfectly. I worry I did poorly on many of them. Did I do OK?"

"Well, it's hard to say right now. It will take me a while to score all of your tests. Remember, we are comparing your scores to other people your age and with your educational background."

"OK, I understand. I need to wait until I come back for the results."

Neuropsychological testing consists of a variety of tests. Each test is designed to measure a different aspect of thinking or memory that, in turn, is performed by a specific network of brain regions. In this way the different parts of the neuropsychological evaluation can tell us how different parts of the brain are doing—which are functioning well and which are impaired. Since different disorders disrupt different brain regions, knowing which brain regions are healthy and which are impaired can help determine what disorder may be affecting the brain. For example, tests that require memorizing a story or list of words evaluate the memory system. We discussed in earlier chapters that the memory system relies upon a network that includes the following: the frontal lobes helping to organize, store, and retrieve memories; the hippocampus that binds and stores new memories; and the cortex that stores older memories. So if you have trouble with tests of memory for new information, we want to know whether it is your frontal lobes or your hippocampus that is not functioning properly. Some of the additional tests help answer this question. Each neuropsychological evaluation including the tests given is a bit different depending upon the individual's symptoms, the different disorders being considered, as well as his or her background, age, and education.

SUMMARY

In this chapter we learned some of the common reasons that someone might need special tests and evaluations of memory beyond what is typically done in a primary care practice. We also learned about what neuropsychologists do and how they can help figure out whether your memory is normal or not—and if not, why not. If you have had either very few or many years of education, if you have a learning disability, if you come from a different culture, or if you have a long-standing psychiatric or other disorder affecting thinking or memory, it may be particularly important for you to have an evaluation with a neuropsychologist to help assess your memory. Lastly, if you are concerned about your memory, get it checked out. Don't wait for memory problems to become disabling.

Let's consider some examples to illustrate what we learned in this chapter.

- You've always been able to look at your calendar in the morning and remember your schedule for the day. Now you find that you need to bring your calendar with you so you don't forget any appointments. Is that just part of getting older?
  o Needing more effort in daily activities that require thinking and memory—such as using calendars, notes, reminders, Google Maps printouts, or a GPS device more than you used to—could be a part of normal aging, but it could also be the first sign of memory loss.

o Bottom line: If you find you need significantly more time and effort for routine activities that rely on thinking and memory, it is a good idea to get your memory checked out.

- You're a sixty-seven-year-old professional and you notice that you are having much more difficulty remembering the information that your clients tell you. You see your primary care physician, who gives you a five-minute quiz of your thinking and memory. You score in the normal range on the quiz. Should you be reassured that your memory is normal?
  o No. If you are very bright or highly educated and you are worried that you have a problem, a neuropsychological evaluation is necessary to evaluate your thinking and memory.
- You never did well in school. You've always wondered if you have a learning disability, such as dyslexia or attention-deficit/hyperactivity disorder. As you've become older, you've been having more trouble with your memory. Your regular doctor gives you a brief test of your thinking and memory. You find you have the same difficulties that you did on tests in school. You score in the impaired range, and your doctor diagnoses you with dementia. Should you ask to see a specialist?
  o Yes. It is difficult to distinguish some types of learning disabilities from early signs of a memory disorder by a brief screening test alone. A neuropsychological evaluation can help to distinguish problems due to long-standing learning disabilities versus those due to a memory disorder.
- You mention to your regular doctor that you are having memory problems, and she refers you to a memory specialist. When you get to the clinic, you find the memory specialist is a psychiatrist. Does that mean your regular doctor thinks you are depressed or crazy or that the memory problems are just "in your head?"
  o Not at all. Memory specialists may be psychiatrists or geriatricians in addition to neurologists and neuropsychologists.
  o Psychiatrists are physicians who have specialized training in disorders of the mind and behavior.
  o Geriatricians are physicians who have first studied internal medicine and then further specialized in disorders of aging.

- You're concerned about your memory, and you have an appointment with a memory specialist. When you made the appointment, they asked you to bring a family member or close friend with you, but you don't want to because you haven't told anyone about your concerns. Do you need to bring someone with you?
  o Someone who knows you well will have a good perspective on whether your memory has changed over time and also remind you of specific instances of memory lapses that you may not recall. If you really don't want anyone to come with you to the appointment, however, it is better to go by yourself than not to go at all.

With the conclusion of this chapter, we have finished Step 2: Determine If Your Memory Is Normal, and you now understand the typical symptoms of Alzheimer's disease, the most common cause of memory loss. We've also discussed the components of a basic memory evaluation that your primary care provider can give you, when a memory specialist is needed, and the role of a neuropsychologist in specialized memory evaluations. We're now ready to turn to the different causes of memory loss in Step 3: Understand Your Memory Loss.

Note: If after going through Steps 1 and 2 you are confident that your memory is normal for your age, and you would like to go directly to what you can do to keep your memory normal and strengthen it, feel free to jump directly to Step 5: Modify Your Lifestyle and Step 6: Strengthen Your Memory.

Step 3

UNDERSTAND YOUR MEMORY LOSS

In Steps 1 and 2 we learned about how to distinguish memory loss that is common and normal in aging from memory loss that could suggest Alzheimer's disease or another disorder. We also learned about the basic parts of an evaluation that are needed to sort out the cause of memory loss and when a specialized evaluation is required. In Step 3 we will learn more about the different causes of memory loss, including Alzheimer's disease, vascular dementia, and dementia with Lewy bodies, as well as those causes of memory loss that are reversible. We'll also discuss what the terms "dementia," "mild cognitive impairment," and "subjective cognitive decline" mean.

6

Will My Memory Get Better?

Which Causes of Memory Loss Are Reversible?

In this chapter we will review many common—and in some cases reversible—causes of memory loss that your doctor should consider as part of your evaluation for memory loss.

NEUROLOGISTS DIAGNOSE AND TREAT BRAIN DISORDERS

When we last left Sue, she had just finished her pencil-and-paper neuropsychological testing. Two weeks have passed, she has had her MRI scan and blood taken, and she and her husband, John, are meeting with the neurologist in his office at the memory center.

"As a neurologist, my role in this evaluation is to look for medical and neurological disorders that can cause problems with thinking and memory. I've spoken with our neuropsychologist, so I'm up to speed on what you discussed with her. I'd like to begin by going over your medical history, and then we'll do a brief physical and neurological exam—listen to your heart and lungs, tap on your reflexes, that sort of thing. After that, we'll review your laboratory studies and your MRI scan together to see what information they can tell us. Then I'll step out for a minute, and the neuropsychologist and I will put our heads together—I'll focus on the medical and neurological side of things, she'll focus on the cognitive and psychological side of things—and we'll see if we can figure out what, if anything, is wrong with your memory and, most importantly, what we can do to make things better. We will give you our joint opinion right afterwards. How does that sound?"

"It sounds great," Sue says, trying to hide her nervousness.

Neurologists are medical doctors who specialize in the diagnosis and treatment of disorders of the brain and other parts of the nervous system. When evaluating a patient for a memory disorder, they are on the lookout for anything that could be interfering with memory as they are going through a person's medical history, current medications, personal habits, lifestyle factors, family history, physical and neurological exam, blood work, and brain imaging studies. Note that although a straightforward memory evaluation does not require a neurologist or other specialist, if the evaluation is complicated, or if a routine evaluation does not yield an answer, seeing a neurologist can be helpful. Some but not all neurologists specialize in memory disorders, so if you are going to see one for your memory, make sure that the neurologist has been trained in memory disorders.

MEDICATION SIDE EFFECTS CAN IMPAIR MEMORY

"I'd like to start by reviewing your medical history. I have the most recent note from your primary care doctor in front of me. The only medical problems listed here are high blood pressure and high cholesterol, is that right?"

"Yes, I take medications for those," Sue responds.

"Right, lisinopril and simvastatin, correct?"

"Yes, that's right."

"Any other medications?"

"No, just those plus a multivitamin."

"Any other over-the-counter medications?"

"Ibuprofen if I have a headache, and over-the-counter sleeping medications if I'm having trouble sleeping."

"How often do you have trouble sleeping?"

"Oh, maybe three or four nights a week."

"I'd like to talk about your sleep in detail on another day. But today I just want to emphasize that those over-the-counter sleep medicines you're taking can actually impair your memory for a day or two after you take them."

"Over-the-counter sleep medicines can impair my memory the next day?" Sue asks with surprise.

"Yes, because of the antihistamines that are in them. The bottom line is that it isn't a problem to take an over-the-counter sleeping medicine once or twice a month if you are having trouble sleeping, but three or four times a week is definitely enough to impair your memory."

"OK," Sue responds hesitantly. "I'll try to only take the over-the-counter sleeping medicine once or twice a month."

One of the most common causes of memory impairment are the side effects of medications, whether prescription or over-the-counter. Any medication that makes you sleepy or comes with the warning "don't operate heavy machinery with this medication" is likely to cause problems with thinking and memory. The most common medications we see in our practices that may impair memory include most sleeping medications (whether over-the-counter or prescription), many cold and allergy medications, many anxiety medications, many prescription pain medications (which often contain morphine or a similar drug), many muscle relaxants, and many of the medications to help with incontinence. If you are taking one or more of these types of medications, that doesn't mean that they are necessarily causing your memory problems, only that you should talk with your doctor about that possibility. Also, even if a medication you are taking is interfering with your memory, it may be important for you to take it for your overall health. But it is still good to understand if a medication is the cause of your memory difficulties, even if you need to keep taking that medication. Lastly, you should always speak with your doctor if you want to stop a medication. Suddenly stopping a medication can cause very serious problems—seizures are one of many side effects that could occur if you stop some of these medications abruptly without reducing the amount of medication slowly.

Classes of Medications That May Interfere with Memory

(See Appendix for more information and for lists of specific medications.)

- Anticholinergic antidepressants
- Antihistamines in cold, flu, and allergy medications
- Antipsychotics
- Anxiety medications: benzodiazepines
- Dizziness and vertigo medications
- Incontinence medications: antispasmodics
- Migraine medications
- Muscle relaxants
- Narcotics opioids
- Nausea, stomach, and bowel medications
- Seizure medications: anticonvulsants
- Sleep medications
- Tremor medications
- Some herbal remedies

Note: If you are taking a medication in one of these classes, you should speak with your doctor about it. Never stop taking a prescribed medication without consulting your doctor.

CHOLESTEROL-LOWERING MEDICATIONS DO NOT CAUSE MEMORY PROBLEMS

You may notice that cholesterol-lowering medications, also called "statins," are not on the list of medications that can cause memory problems. Although there are conflicting claims in the medical literature, we do not believe that statin medications cause memory problems. The best evidence for this view comes from a study that evaluated whether statin medications could actually improve memory. The carefully conducted study found that statins do not improve memory, but neither do they impair memory. The bottom line is that if you are taking a statin medication prescribed by your doctor to lower your cholesterol, we recommend that you continue taking this medication.

MEMORY COMPLAINTS ARE COMMON AROUND THE TIME OF MENOPAUSE

"OK," continues the neurologist, "I've got a few more questions for you. Have you had any major surgeries?"

"No, other than a C-section with the birth of my daughter."

"Speaking of children, when did you go through menopause?"

"Around when I was forty-nine or fifty."

"Did you notice any memory problems at that time?"

"You know, I did, but so did all of my friends who were going through menopause at that time, so I didn't worry about it."

We see many middle-aged women in our practices who noticed a change in their memory corresponding to the time when they were beginning to go through menopause. It is uncertain, however, whether the menopausal changes in estrogen and progesterone are causing the changes in memory, or whether it is just a coincidence because many people around middle age begin to notice a change in their memory. The scientific literature on this topic is unclear. What is clear, however, is that hormone replacement therapy in postmenopausal women does not help cognition or reduce the risk of developing cognitive problems in the future.

ILLEGAL DRUGS CAN DAMAGE THE BRAIN, IMPAIRING THINKING AND MEMORY

"Do you smoke or have you smoked cigarettes?"

"I confess I tried them in college, but nothing more than that."

"Sounds good—we don't count those," he says with a smile. "Have you ever abused any prescription drugs or used illegal drugs?"

"No, nothing like that," Sue answers.

Illegal drugs impair thinking and memory, and many damage the brain—some of them permanently. Cocaine can cause strokes which may permanently damage the brain. Ecstasy decreases the function of the hippocampus and impairs memory even in users who have stopped for a week, with some studies finding a relationship between the degree of impairment in thinking and memory and total lifetime ingestion of ecstasy. Psychedelic drugs (such as lysergic acid diethylamide, better known as LSD) impair memory while being used, with higher doses causing greater impairment. Heroin, morphine, and other similar drugs impair frontal lobe function while in your body, making it difficult for you to store and retrieve memories.

Bottom line: if you are concerned about your memory, don't use illegal drugs. If you have used illegal drugs in the past and are trying to determine if they are the cause of your memory problems now, speaking with your doctor would be the right place to start.

CANNABIS (MARIJUANA) USE CAN IMPAIR THINKING AND MEMORY

Studies of frequent cannabis users have found both impairment in memory and a decrease in the size of the hippocampus. The good news, however, is that when individuals stopped using cannabis for one month, their thinking and memory showed a notable improvement.

CANNABIDIOL (CBD) DOES NOT IMPAIR MEMORY

Two of the many compounds in cannabis are Δ9-tetrahydrocannabinol and cannabidiol, known better as THC and CBD, respectively. It is primarily intoxication with THC that produces the subjective feeling of being "stoned" and impairs memory. CBD, on the other hand, does not appear to impair memory. In fact, some studies found that greater levels of CBD in cannabis can partially compensate for the memory-impairing effects of THC. Studies have not observed memory impairment when CBD alone was used.

ALCOHOL IMPAIRS THINKING AND MEMORY

"OK, how many alcoholic drinks do you have a week, if a drink is twelve ounces of beer, five ounces of wine, or one-and-a-half ounces of liquor?"

"About ten to twelve," Sue calculates. "I have a glass of wine or two with dinner, and I might have a cocktail as well if we go out to a restaurant."

"So, that's a bit more than is recommended. The guidelines, based upon good scientific studies, recommend that both women and men over the age of sixty-five have no more than one or two drinks per day, and no more than seven drinks per week. In addition, even a single drink will impair your ability to form and store new memories. So, if you're meeting new people at a cocktail party and you want to remember their names, my suggestion is to have a nonalcoholic drink.

The good news is that if you are in the habit of having a glass of wine with dinner, as long as you limit it to the recommended amount, it won't cause any permanent damage to the brain."

"Damage? Drinking alcohol can cause brain damage?" John asks.

"Absolutely. Drinking too much alcohol can cause damage to the brain in many different ways. First, alcohol can cause direct damage to the brain's frontal lobes. Second, many people who drink too much alcohol end up falling and hitting their heads, which can further cause damage to the frontal lobes and other parts of the brain. And last but not least, when people are drinking too much alcohol, they sometimes don't eat properly. If this combination of drinking alcohol and poor eating goes on too long, there can be an irreversible memory disorder that develops."

"Wow, I had no idea that alcohol could be so dangerous," John says, somewhat stunned by this news. "No more than two drinks a day, seven drinks a week for me."

Having on average one drink per day is not thought to be harmful. When people drink more than that, however, it can lead not only to impairments in thinking and memory but even permanent brain damage. The frontal lobes can be impaired by alcohol both temporarily and—with continued excess—permanently. Because the frontal lobes are important for learning new information as well as recalling previously learned information, drinking alcohol can make it more difficult to store and retrieve memories. In fact, even a single drink, while not harmful, can still make it more difficult to store and retrieve memories.

Does alcohol affect your memory, even in the recommended amount? There's an easy way to find out. Simply try abstaining from alcohol for two weeks. You may not notice any difference, but you may find an improvement in your thinking and memory.

When alcohol use is heavy (several times the recommended amount) for a prolonged period of time and there is also poor nutrition, specifically a lack of the vitamin B_1 (thiamine), damage to the brain can occur, permanently impairing memory. If severe, it's called Korsakoff's amnesia. Although the condition was once thought to be rare, we now know that many people who have had periods in their lives when they drank heavily have some damage to their brain causing impaired memory. Vitamin B_1 can be found in fish, pork, sunflower seeds, wheat bread, green peas, and many other foods, so its deficiency is uncommon in individuals who are not malnourished. If you think your memory problems could be due to drinking, it is absolutely critical that you abstain from alcohol so as not to make the problem worse.

FAMILY HISTORY CAN INCREASE THE RISK OF ALZHEIMER'S DISEASE

"Anyone in your family with memory problems, Alzheimer's disease, dementia, senility, hardening of the arteries, or a psychiatric disorder late in life?"

"No one had Alzheimer's that I know of. My father died around age eighty-five, I think of a heart attack, but he had memory problems the last few years," Sue answers. "Toward the end he didn't know any of our names. His doctor told us it was senility.

My mother died of lung cancer when she was seventy-two. She didn't have any problems with her memory."

"Anyone else in your family with memory problems?"

"My grandmother, my father's mother, also had memory problems in her late eighties. She lived with us at that time, and I remember that she used to think I was one of her children. I think they called it 'hardening of the arteries.' I confess I don't even know what 'senility' and 'hardening of the arteries' mean."

"Senility is an older term meaning that someone has impaired thinking and memory due to old age. Physicians used to be concerned about problems with thinking and memory only when they happened to people who were younger than age sixty-five. If you were in your eighties, like your father, they just called it senility."

"Is senility a disease?"

"No, it is not a disease, but most people who were given that diagnosis had one or more brain diseases affecting their thinking and memory."

"Like Alzheimer's?" Sue asks.

"Yes. Alzheimer's is the most common disease of aging that affects thinking and memory. So you're right that most people who were told they had senility actually had Alzheimer's disease."

"What about hardening of the arteries?"

"That's an older term meaning atherosclerosis, when cholesterol builds up in the arteries."

"How would that explain memory loss?"

"The idea is that the 'hardening of the arteries' would lead to strokes, and the strokes would lead to memory loss."

"But I don't think my grandmother had any strokes."

"At the time your grandmother was diagnosed, they used to think that strokes were the cause of almost all memory problems, so whenever someone had memory problems, they called it, 'hardening of the arteries,' whether the person had ever had a known stroke or not."

"So what do you think was causing my grandmother's memory problems?" Sue asks.

"Well, if your grandmother had a progressive disorder of memory that started in her eighties and led to her not recognizing people and thinking that you were one of her children, again Alzheimer's is the most likely disease that would cause those problems."

Sue thought about what she had just learned. "So let me just make sure I understand correctly. You're saying that it is likely that my father and grandmother did have Alzheimer's disease?"

"That's correct."

"Does that mean it is likely that I have it, too?" Sue asks with intensity.

"Let's not get ahead of ourselves. With a family history of it, the chance that your memory problems are due to Alzheimer's disease is about two to four times more likely than if you didn't have a family history of it. But Alzheimer's disease is common as we age, so in a very real sense everyone is at risk, family history or not. There are also many other things that we are investigating that could be causing your memory problems—and many of these things are reversible."

Alzheimer's disease is the most common disorder affecting thinking and memory in old age. However, this fact has only been recognized within the past thirty to forty years. Before then, when individuals showed memory loss late in life, it was often attributed to strokes (typically called "hardening of the arteries") or just old age, when the term "senility" was often used. Because Alzheimer's is so common in aging, we are all at risk for developing the disease. If you have a family history of memory problems that sound like Alzheimer's disease in a parent or a sibling, the risk of Alzheimer's disease does rise, such that it becomes two to four times more likely that the cause of your memory problems is due to Alzheimer's rather than something else. But there is certainly a large proportion of people with a family history of Alzheimer's who never develop the disease themselves.

ANXIETY AND DEPRESSION CAN AFFECT MEMORY

"OK, I understand," sighs Sue, looking sad. "I know that we're in the middle of the evaluation and I'll try to be patient. I'm just a bit worried."

"I understand. Let me step back from my questions for one minute. There is no doubt that it is never good to have memory problems. But if you have to have them, now is a better time than ever before. As the neuropsychologist and I will be explaining to you in detail later, there is quite a lot that we can do to help memory problems right now, and there are even more treatments that are being developed. Hang in there just a bit longer as we work with you to sort out what's going on."

"OK, I'll hang in there," Sue says, trying to put on a good face but obviously a bit upset.

"I can see that you're worried about your memory. Let's chat for a minute about your mood. How are you feeling?"

"In general I'm feeling fine, as long as I'm not focused on my memory," Sue replies.

"I can vouch for that," John says, jumping in. "But I have been concerned that Sue has become more and more focused on her memory, such that she is often anxious or sad."

"OK. I always ask about mood because depression and anxiety can actually cause memory problems," the neurologist explains.

"Really?" Sue asks.

"Yes. When people are anxious, they are often preoccupied, thinking about whatever they are anxious about. And when you're thinking about one thing—say that you are worried about your memory—it is difficult to be paying attention to something else. In addition, when we are anxious, our body produces chemicals that put us in that 'fight or flight' mode."

"You mean as if we were facing a tiger or something?" John asks.

"Yes, exactly. The problem is that although the 'fight or flight' mode might be helpful if we are facing a tiger, it is of no use at all when we are facing something like being anxious about a meeting we have next week. All those chemicals released when we are anxious may make it more difficult for us to pay attention, and if we cannot pay attention to something we cannot remember it well."

"That makes sense," Sue agrees.

"It's a similar story with depression. We may be preoccupied with something that is making us sad, and even if we are not, there are chemical changes in the brain that make it difficult for us to concentrate and learn new things."

Anxiety and depression both affect memory. They impair attention and frontal lobe function and, as you know from Steps 1 and 2, that means that anxiety and depression impair the frontal lobes' ability to facilitate the storage and retrieval of information. Because older memories are, in general, the hardest ones to retrieve, and because people with depression have less energy, one characteristic of depression is difficulty retrieving older memories. Note that, as we learned in Step 2, Chapter 4, this pattern is the opposite of that of Alzheimer's disease, when new memories are most affected and older memories are best preserved.

Despite these different patterns, it is sometimes difficult to sort out when depression and anxiety are causing memory problems versus when they are simply normal reactions to worrying about memory problems that are actually caused by something else. Are you having some difficulty with these or other emotions or psychological symptoms? We'll be discussing different ways to cope with these feelings in detail in Step 4, Chapter 12.

HEAD INJURIES AND CHRONIC TRAUMATIC ENCEPHALOPATHY CAN IMPAIR THINKING AND MEMORY

"OK, now I'm going to go through a long list of different symptoms and disorders. Please let me know if you have ever had trouble with any of these."

The neurologist proceeds to ask about whether Sue had ever had a brain infection such as meningitis or encephalitis; a head injury in which she lost consciousness; repetitive mild head injuries from contact sports such as field hockey, lacrosse, or downhill skiing; a stroke or a stroke warning sign, such as sudden weakness or numbness of an arm or a leg, sudden loss of vision, sudden loss of speech; a seizure or convulsion; her eyes playing tricks on her such that she saw people or animals that were not there, like visual hallucinations; trouble walking; falls; a tremor or shaking of the hands or other body part; any major psychiatric problems earlier in life such as major depression or bipolar disease; found any ticks on her body or had a rash that looked like a circle or a bull's eye; or incontinence of bowel or bladder such that she didn't make it to the bathroom on time. Sue responds "no" to each of them.

Head injuries can cause memory loss in at least two different ways. When the head injury first occurs from, for example, a car accident, the brain can be damaged directly when the head hits the windshield or other rigid object. The memory loss, difficulty paying attention, and other symptoms of the brain damage are typically at their worst right after the injury. The symptoms almost always improve over the next two years, although the thinking and memory may not reach the levels that they did prior to the injury.

The second way that head injuries can cause memory loss is in the way that some professional boxers and football players have developed memory loss. We now know that if someone has many small but violent hits to the head—whether or not these hits cause a concussion—the individual may develop a progressive brain disorder that becomes worse over time. This disorder is called chronic traumatic encephalopathy, or CTE for short. If you played football in college, experienced intimate partner violence, or experienced other activities in which you had many violent blows to the head, you should discuss with your doctor whether you may be developing chronic traumatic encephalopathy.

SEIZURES MAY CAUSE PERIODS OF UNRESPONSIVENESS

Sometimes seizures are obvious, as when someone loses consciousness, has a whole-body convulsion, and their arms and legs become stiff and jerk for about minute or so. However there are other types of seizures in which individuals simply "space out" and are unresponsive for a couple of seconds up to a minute or so. These mini-seizures, sometimes called "petit mal," "focal," or "complex partial" seizures, can interfere with memory formation and retrieval. Although they are not a common cause of memory loss, they are treatable with medications and, if untreated, can cause other problems such as accidents if they occur when driving. If people have told you that you have periods of time when you "space out" and don't respond, you should discuss with your doctor whether you should be evaluated for seizures.

LYME DISEASE AND OTHER INFECTIONS CAN CAUSE MEMORY LOSS

There are many infections that can cause trouble with thinking and memory, including diseases spread by ticks such as Lyme disease and Rocky Mountain spotted fever. If you live in an area where these or other such diseases are common and you spend time outdoors in the woods or you have found a tick on you, you should speak with your doctor about getting tested for one of these treatable diseases.

There are many other treatable infectious diseases that can interfere with thinking and memory. If you are having any symptoms of infection such as fever, cough, night sweats, chills, or muscle aches, you should see your doctor right away to find out if you have a treatable infection. Finally, if you think it is possible that you have contracted a sexually transmitted disease, make sure you mention it to your doctor. Two sexually transmitted diseases, syphilis and HIV, may first become noticeable because of thinking and memory difficulties.

A NEUROLOGICAL EXAM LOOKS FOR BRAIN AND NERVOUS SYSTEM DISORDERS

"Now I'd like to move to the physical and neurological exam. The only undressing you need to do is to take off your shoes and socks."

"Isn't that the wrong end to be examining?" John asks, smiling.

"I know, I know, everyone thinks it's funny that a brain doctor wants to look at the feet, but you'll see that I examine all of the muscles and nerves from head to toe."

Sue climbs on the exam table and sits comfortably with her legs dangling as the neurologist begins to examine her. Some parts of the exam she is familiar with: he listens to her heart and lungs, tests her vision and hearing, shines a light and looks in her eyes, has her stick out her tongue and say "ahh," and pushes on her belly. Other parts of the exam are new to her. He listens with his stethoscope on each side of her neck. He asks her to follow his finger all over with her eyes, explaining he is looking at how her eyes move. Wiggling his fingers on the left, right, top, and bottom of her vision, he determines how well she can see out of the corners of her eyes. He next explains that he is going to examine her muscles, and starts by having her raise her eyebrows, close her eyes tight, and smile. Then he tests her strength in her arms and legs—including her fingers and toes. He examines her sensation by asking whether she can feel a light touch on her face, arms, legs, fingers, and toes, and then whether she can feel the coolness of a metal tuning fork in those same areas.

The neurologist continues, now using a reflex hammer to tap on her lips, arms, elbows, knees, and ankles. Sue never knew she had so many reflexes! He then scratches the bottom of her feet with the pointed end of the hammer. Taking her hands in his, he next moves them around, looking at how easily he can move them. He then asks her to make a pointing finger and go back and forth touching his finger and her nose as he moves his finger around. He next has her flip each hand—palm up and then palm down—quickly. Lastly, he asks her to stand up, put her feet together, put her hands out palm side up, close her eyes, and keep standing.

"It's a little balance test," he says. Sue passes the balance test and he continues, "OK, all that looks fine. You can go ahead and put your shoes and socks back on."

Noting that Sue is looking amused, he smiles back and explains, "I know that many of these tests may seem quite silly, but they all help me to see how the different parts of your brain and your nervous system are working."

In addition to conducting the usual parts of a physical examination that most physicians do, a neurologist also performs a specialized neurological exam to look for any problems with the brain or nervous system. This specialized exam can look for problems such as strokes, tumors, Parkinson's disease, tremors, multiple sclerosis, and many other disorders that could give a clue to the cause of thinking and memory problems. Vision and hearing are always evaluated because if one cannot see or hear well, it won't be possible to remember information coming in through the eyes and ears.

THYROID DISORDERS ARE COMMON

"OK, now let's review the results from your blood draw. There are a few abnormalities to discuss."

Sue and John look up, waiting for him to continue.

"The first is that the thyroid screening test that we ran is abnormal, and I want you to follow up with your primary doctor. You may be hypothyroid, meaning that your thyroid gland isn't producing enough hormone for your body."

"What does the thyroid do?" Sue asks.

"The thyroid gland produces thyroid hormone that helps regulate the metabolism of just about every system in your body, making sure that they are all running at the right speed. So if your thyroid levels are low, it can cause difficulty concentrating. Having low thyroid hormone is very common in older adults, which is why we test for it. And don't worry, we can easily treat it by simply giving you more thyroid hormone in a pill."

Screening for thyroid disorders with a simple blood test is part of any evaluation for memory problems. Abnormal thyroid hormone levels may cause impaired memory, difficulty concentrating, irritability, mood instability, restlessness, and confusion.

DEFICIENCIES OF VITAMINS B_{12} AND D ARE COMMON

"I'm so glad that the thyroid problem is easy to treat," Sue says. "What else was abnormal?"

"Two of your vitamin levels were low: B_{12} and D."

"Are they important?" asks Sue.

"Yes. If your vitamin B$_{12}$ level is low, it can cause many neurological issues, including problems with thinking and memory, along with fatigue, sleepiness, and depression. To treat it, we'll start by simply having you take over-the-counter vitamin B$_{12}$ pills, and we will recheck your levels in a couple of months. If it is still low, you can get B$_{12}$ shots, as some people cannot absorb B$_{12}$ in pill form."

"What about vitamin D?"

"We know that vitamin D is important for bones and muscles, and it may be important for thinking and memory as well. So I recommend that you take vitamin D pills along with the B$_{12}$."

A deficiency of vitamin B$_{12}$ can cause very serious problems, including difficulties with thinking, memory, and mood, and so it should always be checked as part of a memory evaluation.

A deficiency of vitamin D has not been proven to cause memory loss, but a strong correlation has been found between low vitamin D levels and dementia. We therefore recommend either having your vitamin D levels checked or speaking with your doctor about simply taking 2,000 IU of over-the-counter vitamin D$_3$ daily. (See also Step 5, Chapter 14.)

DIABETES AND OTHER MEDICAL ISSUES CAN IMPAIR THINKING AND MEMORY

Many medical disorders can impair thinking and memory, so your doctor should evaluate you for common medical problems with a physical exam and some laboratory studies. Diabetes deserves special mention because it can cause memory problems in several ways. First, diabetes is a risk factor for strokes that can cause memory trouble. Second, when the levels of the blood sugar rise too high or go too low, there can be episodes of confusion and memory loss. Lastly, the hippocampus and other parts of the brain can be permanently damaged if control of diabetes is too strict and blood sugars are repeatedly dropping to dangerously low levels.

BRAIN IMAGING STUDIES CAN SHOW ATROPHY, STROKES, TUMORS, AND OTHER ABNORMALITIES

"OK, let's take a look at your MRI scan together now," the neurologist says, turning a large monitor on his desk so Sue can see. "Many parts of your brain look great—better than average, in fact, for your age. There are, however, a couple of parts I want to show you. The first is this part of your temporal lobe, next to the temples of your head, just behind your eyes. Do you see that there is more black space around the grey brain? That suggests that there is some shrinkage. Now everyone your age has some shrinking here, but you have a bit more than I would expect."

"What does that part of the brain do?" Sue asks.

"It is involved with naming, particularly the names of people."

"Well, that doesn't surprise me . . . as you know, I'm having some trouble with people's names."

"Next I want to point out these crescent-shaped structures on the inside portion of the brain. This is your hippocampus—one on each side—where new memories are stored. Do you see the black space around it? Again, that suggests to me that they have shrunken up a bit."

"Well, that fits with my memory problems."

"Right. Here are your frontal lobes, which look great. They are in charge of a lot of things, including organizing and planning for the future, focusing attention, and doing complicated activities."

"Well, it's good that something in my brain isn't shrinking!"

"There is just one other area that I want to point out. Do you see this area in the back of the brain?"

"Yes, and I can already see the large black areas around the thin grey parts of the brain."

"Correct. These are your parietal lobes. They help you pay attention and are also important for navigating through the world, such as planning a route."

"I do find that I need to spend a bit more time thinking of how I am going to go from one place to another," Sue says.

"So, in summary, there is some shrinkage of your temporal and parietal lobes, as well as the hippocampus. The rest of your brain looks great, and I didn't see any strokes, bleeding, tumors, fluid collections, or other problems."

"Well, that's a relief," Sue says. "But what does it mean that those three areas of the brain have shrunken?"

"It might not mean anything, but I confess that we do often see that pattern of shrinkage in people who have Alzheimer's disease."

"Are you saying that I have Alzheimer's disease?" asks Sue, sounding concerned.

John looks at Sue and then the neurologist, waiting for an answer.

"No, not at all. You cannot diagnose Alzheimer's disease just by looking at the scan. That's why we do the whole evaluation. In just a minute I'm going to speak with our neuropsychologist, and we are going to put our heads together and look at all of the different parts of the evaluation to try to understand the cause of your memory difficulties."

"OK, I understand. You need to interpret the pattern of shrinkage in context," Sue remarks.

"Exactly."

An MRI or CT scan can detect brain disorders such as strokes, bleeds, tumors, fluid collections, multiple sclerosis, some infections, and many other disorders. You can also see patterns of brain atrophy (shrinkage) that may be common in one or another brain disease. However, patterns of brain atrophy are just one piece of evidence that can be evaluated when your doctor is making a diagnosis. You cannot know for sure that someone does or does not have a particular brain disease affecting memory just by looking at a brain imaging scan.

SUMMARY

In this chapter we learned some of the most common causes of memory loss that are reversible, including medication side effects, vitamin deficiencies, alcohol use, thyroid disorders, depression, and anxiety. We also learned about what neurologists do and—although not necessarily routine—how they can participate in a memory evaluation. Lastly, we learned a bit about some additional parts of the brain and what information a brain imaging study (such as an MRI or CT scan) can show us.

Let's consider some examples to illustrate what we learned in this chapter.

- Ever since you started a new prescription medication, you have felt tired and your thinking has been foggy. Should you stop the medication and see if your thinking improves?
  o Only after speaking with your doctor! Although medications are a common cause of memory problems, you should never stop a prescription medication without speaking to your doctor first.
- You have begun to notice memory problems, and you are worried they could represent something bad, such as Alzheimer's disease or a brain tumor. You are feeling very anxious. Are the memory problems likely related to the anxiety?
  o When one has memory problems along with anxiety or depression, it can be difficult to determine which problem is primary and which may be secondary. You should discuss your concerns about memory and depression or anxiety with your doctor.
- You have been feeling "run-down" lately. Your mood is fine, you're getting plenty of sleep, but you just don't have any energy. What should you do?
  o Speak with your doctor about these symptoms. They could be due to low thyroid hormone, which is more common as we get older.
- For the past month you have been having chills, and you find your pajamas wet with sweat when you wake up. What should you do?

o Speak with your doctor about these symptoms. They may be related to an infection, which can be treated.

- Your memory has been worse for the past month, about the same time that you have noticed that you are having more trouble hearing what people are saying to you. What should you do?
  o If you cannot hear what people are saying to you, you won't be able to remember it. Discuss having your hearing evaluated with your doctor. If you have a hearing aid, make sure that it is functioning properly.

- For some things your memory is excellent, but for other things it is terrible. Your spouse tells you that you seem to be "spacing out," sometimes in the middle of a sentence. You're unaware of these episodes and are quite sure that you are not just daydreaming. What should you do?
  o Seizures are an unusual cause of memory problems, but they are both serious and treatable. If you are having these kinds of "spacing-out" episodes, you should discuss them with your doctor.

- You notice that you don't remember the prior evening well if you had a couple of drinks that night.
  o Everyone has more trouble remembering events if they have a few drinks, but alcohol is more likely to affect memory in older individuals and in those with memory problems due to any cause. Try abstaining from alcohol for a time to see if that helps.

7

What Are Dementia, Mild Cognitive Impairment, and Subjective Cognitive Decline?

After having considered many causes of cognitive impairment in Chapter 6, in this chapter we will learn what dementia is and what terms are used to indicate intermediate stages between normal aging and dementia.

BRING A FAMILY MEMBER OR CLOSE FRIEND WITH YOU WHEN YOU ARE RECEIVING THE RESULTS OF YOUR EVALUATION

When we last saw Jack, he was in the doctor's office having his memory evaluated. Let's catch up with Jack now as he and his daughter, Sara, are meeting with the doctor to go over the results of his memory evaluation.

"Hi, Jack. How are you doing today?" the doctor asks.

"Nervous, doc, about the results of my tests," Jack replies. "Have you met my daughter, Sara?"

"I don't think so. Nice to meet you, Sara. Thanks for coming in with your father today."

"Nice to meet you as well," Sara responds.

It's always a good idea to have someone with you when you are hearing the results of any medical evaluation. That person can take notes for you, allowing you to focus your full attention on the doctor, the results of the tests, the diagnosis, and the plan for medications or other treatment. And, of course, it is even more important to bring someone with you if you are having trouble with your memory.

DEMENTIA INDICATES IMPAIRMENT OF DAILY FUNCTION DUE TO PROBLEMS WITH THINKING AND MEMORY

"I do have your test results," the doctor continues, "including the questionnaire and the pencil-and-paper tests that we gave you earlier, as well as your blood work and your MRI scan. I want to begin by saying that given the results of the tests and how you are functioning, you don't have dementia."

"That's great! But what kind of disease is dementia?" Jack asks. "I'm worried about Alzheimer's, not dementia."

Sara, taking notes, now also looks up.

"Dementia is not a disease, but is the term we use when there is a loss of one's thinking and memory abilities to the point that one's function is impaired in everyday life. If someone has dementia, they have difficulty living alone and managing their affairs by themselves."

"You mean like trouble bathing and getting dressed?" Jack asks.

"People with dementia may not only have problems like those—which would indicate the moderate stage of dementia—but problems such as difficulty paying bills, doing the shopping, or taking their medications correctly."

"I don't think my dad has problems with those things, do you, Dad?" Sara asks.

"No, not with those things," Jack answers.

"Exactly. It is because you don't have those kind of problems, Jack, that I know you don't have dementia," the doctor explains.

"Well, I'm glad I don't have dementia," Jack says. "I wasn't even worried about it. . . . What causes dementia anyways?"

"Many different disorders can cause dementia. Alzheimer's disease is the most common cause, but one can also have dementia due to strokes (which we call vascular dementia), Parkinson's disease, head injuries, infections, or even vitamin deficiencies. And there are many other causes of dementia as well."

When people have problems with their thinking and memory to the point that they can no longer function independently, they have dementia. People are diagnosed with dementia when three things are present:

- Concern that there has been a prominent decline in thinking and memory by the individual, their family, or their doctor.
- Substantial impairment on tests of thinking and memory.
- The thinking and memory problems interfere with their everyday activities.

They have mild dementia if there is only difficulty doing somewhat complicated daily activities, such as paying bills, shopping, or taking medicines. Difficulties with more basic activities of daily living, such as dressing, bathing, and using the toilet, suggest that the dementia is in the moderate or severe stage.

Activities of Daily Living
Complex activities of daily living
- Performing housework

- Taking medications
- Preparing meals
- Shopping
- Paying bills and managing money

Basic activities of daily living
- Dressing and undressing
- Bathing
- Eating
- Using the toilet
- Controlling bowel and bladder

DEMENTIA CAN BE CAUSED BY MANY DIFFERENT DISORDERS

Dementia is not a disease in itself; it is a condition with many different causes. It is like a headache, which could be due to muscle tension, migraines, a blood clot, or a tumor. Just like a headache, some causes of dementia are relatively benign and easily treatable, whereas other causes are more serious and may have no treatment. Alzheimer's disease is the cause of dementia about 60 percent of the time, which is why people often confuse Alzheimer's disease and dementia. Other common causes of dementia include Parkinson's disease dementia (which is similar to dementia with Lewy bodies), vascular dementia, and frontotemporal dementia. We'll learn about the specific causes of dementia in Step 3, Chapters 8, 9, and 10.

SUBJECTIVE COGNITIVE DECLINE MAY BE A SIGN OF A FUTURE MEMORY DISORDER—BUT NOT ALWAYS

"OK, so if I don't have dementia, is my memory normal?" Jack asks.

"Well, let's talk about that. The first thing I want to note is that you told me that you were concerned about your memory, that it wasn't as good as it used to be. We have learned over the last couple of years that if you notice a decline in your memory and are concerned about it enough to go to your doctor, your chances of having a real memory disorder are somewhat greater than if you are not experiencing any problems—even if your memory testing is completely normal."

"Wait—just because I told you I'm concerned about my memory, are you telling me that it means I have a memory disorder?" Jack interjects.

"No, not at all, but your chances of having a memory disorder are somewhat greater. We typically call this situation when people have noticed memory problems but have tested normally 'subjective cognitive decline.' One way to think about it is that most people know themselves pretty well, so that if they think there is a problem with their memory, they are often correct."

"Does that also mean that many people with this subjective cognitive decline don't end up having disorder?" asks Sara.

"Yes, exactly. We think of subjective cognitive decline as a risk factor for developing a disorder in the future, not a disorder itself, nor a sure sign that a disorder will develop."

If you have noticed that your memory has declined, you are concerned about it enough to see your doctor, and your doctor tested you and told you that your memory is normal, you have "subjective cognitive decline" (sometimes called "subjective cognitive impairment"). Individuals have subjective cognitive decline when:

- They have noticed a decline in thinking or memory (or both) bothersome enough for them to bring it to the attention of their doctor.
- Their performance on tests of thinking and memory is normal.
- Their daily function is normal.

Compared to individuals without concerns about their memory, those with subjective cognitive decline are somewhat more likely to end up with a diagnosable memory disorder over five to ten years.

Does that sound a bit frightening? Please don't be alarmed—by addressing your concerns you are doing the right thing. First, most people with subjective cognitive decline don't end up having a memory disorder or they have something reversible as we discussed in the last chapter, such as a vitamin deficiency or thyroid disorder. You should see your doctor to look for these and other reversible causes. Second, in this book we are going to discuss specific things that you can do today to help improve your memory and make it less likely that you will end up with a memory disorder in the future, including improving your diet and engaging in exercise (Step 5). Lastly, as we will learn in Step 4, even if you do end up being diagnosed with a memory disorder, many good treatments are available—and the benefits of these treatments are greatest when started early. Read on!

IN MILD COGNITIVE IMPAIRMENT THERE IS A DECLINE IN MEMORY OR THINKING, BUT FUNCTION IS NORMAL

"So is that what I've got, Doc, 'subjective cognitive decline'?" Jack asks.

"Do you remember the pencil-and-paper tests that we gave you?"

"Yes . . . mostly. I know I didn't score perfectly on that test," Jack responds.

"Right. On that test you scored 23 out of a possible 30."

"Is that bad?" Sara asks.

"No, it isn't bad, but it is a bit below 26, which is considered the lower end of normal."

"So what does that mean?" Jack asks.

"Because your memory testing was abnormal, it means that you don't have subjective cognitive decline. You have what we call 'mild cognitive impairment.' We use this term when

> you or someone who knows you well has noticed a decline
> in your memory or thinking, there is evidence of this decline
> on pencil-and-paper testing, but your function is essentially
> normal—so it is not dementia."
>
> "Yeah, that fits," agrees Jack. He then continues, sighing, "But
> the only reason that I'm able to do things normally is that
> I need to put in a lot more effort."
>
> "And that is exactly what people with mild cognitive impair-
> ment typically do—they can still do everything they want to
> do; they just need to put in more effort when doing it."

We use the term "mild cognitive impairment" when three things are present:

- A decline in memory or thinking (or both) has been noticed by the individual, their family, or their doctor.
- Impairment—typically mild—is present on tests of thinking and memory.
- Daily function is essentially normal, although activities may require a bit more effort.

Individuals with mild cognitive impairment don't have subjective cognitive decline because there is objective impairment on tests of thinking and memory, and they don't have dementia because their function is normal.

ALTHOUGH MANY PEOPLE WITH MILD COGNITIVE IMPAIRMENT EXPERIENCE A DECLINE IN THINKING AND MEMORY OVER TIME, SOME REMAIN STABLE AND OTHERS IMPROVE

> "OK, I think I understand what 'mild cognitive impairment'
> means," Sara chimes in. "But what about the future? If my

dad has mild cognitive impairment, does that mean his thinking and memory will get worse over time?"

Jack turns his gaze nervously from Sara to the doctor.

"Good question. The answer is that about half of those with mild cognitive impairment do show declines in their thinking and memory over several years and ultimately develop dementia. But that also means that the other half of people diagnosed with mild cognitive impairment do not develop dementia—their thinking and memory either stays stable or returns to normal."

"You mean that there is a chance that my memory will stay the same or actually improve?" Jack asks, the hope evident in his voice.

"Yes, that's exactly what I'm saying."

Approximately 50 percent of individuals with mild cognitive impairment show declines in thinking and memory that leads to dementia, at a rate of about 5 to 15 percent per year. However, that means that the other 50 percent remain stable or improve.

Have you been diagnosed with mild cognitive impairment? The good news is that—even if you don't do anything—there is a good chance that your thinking and memory will stay stable or improve. More importantly, in Steps 4, 5, and 6 we are going to discuss exactly what you can do to improve your memory and make it less likely that you will develop dementia in the future.

MILD COGNITIVE IMPAIRMENT CAN BE CAUSED BY MANY DIFFERENT DISORDERS

"What causes mild cognitive impairment?" Sara asks.

"Many different disorders can cause mild cognitive impairment, just as many different disorders can cause dementia.

> In fact, the list of possible disorders is even longer, and can include things like depression, anxiety, and thyroid disorders, as well as all those things that can cause dementia, such as Alzheimer's disease and strokes."

Like dementia, mild cognitive impairment is not a disease in itself—it is a condition with many different causes. In individuals over the age of sixty-five, Alzheimer's disease is the most common cause of mild cognitive impairment. Other common causes include strokes and Parkinson's disease, as well as depression, anxiety, thyroid disorders, vitamin deficiencies, infections, medication side effects, and medical problems.

SUMMARY

In this chapter we learned some of the basic terminology associated with disorders of thinking and memory. In dementia, there is impairment in daily function caused by substantial impairment of thinking and memory. In mild cognitive impairment, daily function is normal, but there is mild impairment on tests of thinking and memory. In subjective cognitive decline, performance on tests of thinking and memory is normal, although individuals are concerned enough about their memory to bring it to their doctors' attention. We also learned that although none of these terms indicate a specific disorder, Alzheimer's disease is the most common cause of both dementia and mild cognitive impairment.

Let's consider some examples to illustrate what we learned in this chapter.

- You have seen your doctor because you are concerned about your memory. He gives you a memory test, and you score in the normal range. Does that mean you are unlikely to develop a memory disorder in the future?

o If you have concerns about your memory worrisome enough to go to your doctor but you score normally on tests of thinking and memory, you have subjective cognitive decline. People with subjective cognitive decline are somewhat more likely to develop disorders of memory in the future than those who do not have concerns about their memory.

- You've just been diagnosed with mild cognitive impairment. Does that mean you will definitely develop dementia due to Alzheimer's disease in the future?
   o No, although your chances of developing either Alzheimer's disease or another disorder of memory that can lead to dementia are about 50 percent. That also means that you have about a 50 percent chance of your thinking and memory remaining stable or improving.
- Is dementia the same thing as Alzheimer's disease?
   o No. Dementia is a general term indicating that thinking and memory have deteriorated to the point that daily function is impaired. Alzheimer's disease is one of many causes of dementia. Other causes of dementia include strokes, infections, vitamin deficiencies, and other neurologic diseases.
- I'm concerned about my memory but afraid that I will be told I have one of these conditions. If there is something wrong with my memory, can the doctor actually do anything to help me?
   o Yes! Seeing your doctor about your memory concerns is very important. You may have an infection, vitamin deficiency, thyroid disorder, or depression such that, after treatment, your memory may return to normal. In addition, there are medications available to help people with memory disorders that can make a real difference.

8

What Is Alzheimer's Disease?

Now that we understand what the terms "dementia," "mild cognitive impairment," and "subjective cognitive decline" mean, we are ready to learn about the major neurological disorders that lead to these conditions. We will begin with Alzheimer's disease, the most common disorder that causes memory loss in the older adult. We learned about the symptoms of Alzheimer's disease in Step 2, Chapters 3 and 4. In this chapter we'll learn about how Alzheimer's disease damages the brain.

ALZHEIMER'S DISEASE HAS MANY STAGES

When we last saw Sue, she was undergoing her neurological examination. Let's catch up with Sue as she and her husband, John, meet with the neuropsychologist to hear the results of the memory center's comprehensive evaluation.

"OK, so we've put our heads together and now I want to share the results of your cognitive tests, our thoughts about your memory, and our plan of action."

Sue looks at John nervously and then looks back to the neuropsychologist. John smiles supportively at Sue, but his concern shows on his face.

"On your cognitive tests—the pencil-and-paper tests we gave you to evaluate your thinking and memory—you scored a bit lower than we would have expected for someone of your age and education. Now because the impairment in your thinking and memory is quite mild, and you have no problems with your function, the term we use is 'mild cognitive impairment.'"

"Does that mean I have Alzheimer's disease?" Sue asks.

"There are a lot different things that can cause mild cognitive impairment. Alzheimer's is one of them, but there are many other possible causes. Our neurologist and I think that some of the different things that he discussed with you—the sleeping medicine, alcohol, vitamins B_{12} and D, and the low thyroid—either alone or in combination, could explain your performance on the pencil-and-paper memory tests, and the mild difficulty with memory that you have noticed."

"But what about my MRI scan that showed shrinkage in the brain? And what about my family history of Alzheimer's disease, although it was called senility or hardening of the arteries at the time. Doesn't all that mean it is likely that I have Alzheimer's disease?" asks Sue, with concern.

"Although there are a lot of other things to look into, there is no doubt that Alzheimer's is one possible explanation for your mild cognitive impairment."

"I thought Alzheimer's disease was a type of *dementia*," John says, puzzled. "I didn't know it could cause something so mild, like this 'mild cognitive impairment.'"

"Our current understanding is that the Alzheimer's disease process actually starts in the brain a number of years before there are any symptoms at all. As it progresses and thinking and memory begin to be affected—but function in daily life is still normal—Alzheimer's first becomes noticeable as mild cognitive impairment. When the disease advances and daily function is impaired, it has reached the dementia stage. The dementia stage can be divided further into very mild, mild, moderate, and severe stages."

Alzheimer's disease starts in the brain years before any symptoms are noticeable. Over time, when thinking and memory begin to be affected yet day-to-day function is normal, the disease has reached the mild cognitive impairment stage. Only when function is impaired do we refer to it as "Alzheimer's disease dementia." In the very mild stage of dementia, function is just a bit impaired; for example, individuals may no longer be able to perform the complicated activities that they did previously such as remodeling a bathroom or hosting a large dinner party. In the next, mild stage, forgetfulness and other problems with thinking begin to interfere with more routine activities such as cooking, shopping, and paying bills. In the moderate stage daily living activities, including dressing and bathing, become difficult. In the severe stage, people with Alzheimer's have difficulty communicating, recognizing family members, and remaining continent. Even once dementia is present, Alzheimer's disease is a slow process. Without treatment, people with Alzheimer's typically progress from the very mild to the severe stage over a period ranging from four to twelve years.

ALZHEIMER'S IS A BRAIN DISEASE CHARACTERIZED BY AMYLOID PLAQUES AND NEUROFIBRILLARY TANGLES

"What exactly is Alzheimer's disease, anyways?" asks John.

"Alzheimer's is a brain disease in which there is a buildup of an abnormal protein called 'beta-amyloid.' When too much amyloid is present, it forms these clumps that we call 'plaques.' As the disease progresses, 'cleanup cells' in the brain react to the plaques and an inflammatory reaction can occur that causes damage to brain cells and leads to larger plaques. At this point the amyloid plaques interfere with the communication between brain cells and that begins to interfere with brain function."

"So is it these 'amyloid plaques' that cause Alzheimer's disease?" asks Sue.

"That's how we believe it starts. Once the plaques start to injure the brain cells, it causes 'tangles' to form inside the cells. It is these tangles that then kill the brain cells."

In 1906 the psychiatrist Alois Alzheimer looked at brain tissue from one of his patients under a microscope and first saw amyloid plaques and neurofibrillary tangles. We now know that the plaques are a mixture of beta-amyloid, parts of brain cells, as well as other substances found between and outside the cells. Although there is much active research trying to understand the exact relationship between amyloid plaques and cognitive function, one possible link is as follows: when the plaques first form, they don't necessarily cause problems, but once the "cleanup cells" in the brain—part of the brain's immune system—begin to react to the plaques, an inflammatory reaction occurs that disrupts communication between brain cells and interferes with brain function.

Damage to the cells from the plaques causes neurofibrillary tangles to form inside them. We call them "tangles" because they look like tangled string under the microscope. The tangles are composed of parts of the skeleton and nutrient system

Table 8.1 Brain Regions Affected by Alzheimer's Disease and Their Functions

Regions	Functions	Time Affected
Hippocampus	New memory formation and storage	Early
Anterior temporal lobes	Word finding	Early
Parietal lobes	Attention and spatial function	Early
Frontal lobes	Focused attention for learning new information, as well as planning, behavior, and complicated activities	Late

of the dying brain cell, also called a neuron. Ultimately, as Alzheimer's disease progresses, more and more brain cells are damaged by plaques, form tangles, and die.

ALZHEIMER'S DISEASE AFFECTS THE HIPPOCAMPUS, TEMPORAL LOBES, AND PARIETAL LOBES EARLY, AND THE FRONTAL LOBES LATER

"Is that why one can see shrinkage in some areas of the brain, because cells are dying there?" asks John.

"Exactly right," agrees the neuropsychologist. "Alzheimer's disease affects three regions of the brain first: the hippocampus on the inside of the temporal lobes, causing memory loss, particularly for new information; the temporal lobes, causing word-finding difficulties; and the parietal lobes, which can lead to difficulty with attention and finding one's way around. The frontal lobes, involved with planning, behavior, and performing complicated activities, tend to be affected a bit later. So when we look at the brain on an MRI or CT scan, we look to see if there is shrinkage in these regions."

When enough brain cells die in a particular region, that region of the brain no longer functions as well as it did, and atrophy can often be seen on an MRI or CT scan. Table 8.1 lists the brain regions affected by Alzheimer's, their functions, and whether they tend to be affected early or late by the disease.

GENES CAN CAUSE TOO MUCH BETA-AMYLOID TO ACCUMULATE

"Why does beta-amyloid build up in the brain and form plaques in some people and not others?" asks Sue.

"That's a good question," says the neuropsychologist. "Some people have a gene that leads to either overproduction of beta-amyloid or not enough clearance of it. The most common genetic variation associated with Alzheimer's disease is the 'APOE-e4' gene. People with this gene appear to not clear beta-amyloid as quickly as other people do."

"Do we know if my father had this 'APOE-e4' gene? Should I be tested for it?"

"We don't recommend testing for this genetic variation because having it doesn't mean you have Alzheimer's and not having it doesn't mean you don't have Alzheimer's. Approximately half of the people with Alzheimer's disease do have this gene, but the other half do not. It is a risk factor for the disease, not an indication that one will get it for sure."

Although we don't know exactly what the normal function of beta-amyloid is, everyone's brain makes it. It may be involved in fighting off brain infections. Alzheimer's disease develops when too much beta-amyloid accumulates, leading to plaques. We know that some people have genetic differences that cause either too much amyloid to be formed or not enough to be cleared. The most common genetic variation that can lead to Alzheimer's disease is the APOE-e4 gene, which appears to be related to reduced clearance of beta-amyloid. But we do not recommend testing for it, as it cannot determine whether Alzheimer's disease is present or not or whether it will develop in the future.

FAMILY HISTORY OF ALZHEIMER'S DISEASE INCREASES THE CHANCES OF DEVELOPING IT BETWEEN TWOFOLD AND FOURFOLD

There are families in several places in the world (such as Colombia, South America) where a genetic mutation causes beta-amyloid to accumulate leading to young-onset Alzheimer's disease before age sixty-five—and often before age fifty—in nearly 100 percent of those carrying the mutation. But there is no such family history in the majority of individuals who develop late-onset Alzheimer's disease after age sixty-five.

The development of Alzheimer's disease is, unfortunately, very common with age. We are all at risk for it, and the risk grows as we age, approaching 50 percent by age eighty-five. Family history in a parent or sibling does increase the risk of developing Alzheimer's between twofold and fourfold. For example, if the overall risk of developing Alzheimer's disease between ages sixty-five and seventy is about 2.5 percent, the risk without a family history is about 1.5 percent, whereas the risk with a family history is between 3 and 6 percent.

ALZHEIMER'S DISEASE IS MORE COMMON IN WOMEN

"What are the other reasons that people develop Alzheimer's disease besides genes and family history?"

"That is a good question, and one that we don't have a complete answer for," the neuropsychologist says. "Three other things that have been strongly associated with Alzheimer's disease include age, suffering a head injury, and being a woman."

"I'm at risk for Alzheimer's disease just because I'm a woman?"

"Yes, in fact, in the United States about two-thirds of individuals with Alzheimer's disease are women."

"Is that just because women live longer than men?" asks John.

"That's part of the explanation. But there may be other reasons as well. There's a lot of research trying to answer that question."

Of the 6.2 million people in the United States with Alzheimer's disease age sixty-five and older, approximately 3.8 million are women. Part of the reason for this is that Alzheimer's is more common as people age, and women live longer than men. Other explanations are being actively investigated.

HEAD TRAUMA INCREASES THE RISK OF ALZHEIMER'S DISEASE

It has been observed for many years that suffering a head injury puts one at increased risk for developing dementia. Initially it was believed that almost all of the individuals who developed dementia after head injury had Alzheimer's as the cause of their dementia. From more recent studies of boxers and football players, we now know that at least some of these individuals with head injuries—particularly when the head injuries are repetitive—develop chronic traumatic encephalopathy (see Step 3, Chapter 6). But there is no doubt that suffering a head injury also puts one at increased risk for Alzheimer's disease.

ALZHEIMER'S DISEASE IS NOT PART OF NORMAL AGING

"I can't believe that I'm at increased risk for Alzheimer's disease just because I am a woman," Sue exclaims. "And just because I am 80 years old! If Alzheimer's is more and more common as people get older, and age is a risk factor for it, is Alzheimer's just part of normal aging?"

"No. We think of Alzheimer's as one of many diseases that are more common as we get older, such as diabetes, high blood pressure, cancer, and cataracts. We don't consider it part of normal aging."

Given how common Alzheimer's disease is in individuals in their seventies and eighties, it is very reasonable to wonder if Alzheimer's is just part of normal aging. However, there are many people who live into their nineties or even hundreds without developing Alzheimer's disease either clinically or pathologically (when their brains are looked at after death under a microscope). In fact, it is estimated that roughly half of individuals age eighty-five and older do not have Alzheimer's or any other type of dementia. So although Alzheimer's disease is more common with aging, it is not a normal part of it.

EDUCATION AND INTELLIGENCE MAY REDUCE THE RISK OF ALZHEIMER'S DISEASE

"Family history, being a woman, being older . . . it seems like I have all the risk factors. Are there any factors that make my risk of Alzheimer's less likely?" asks Sue.

"Yes, I was actually just going to mention one. The more education you have, the less likely you are to develop Alzheimer's disease. So, because you have a master's degree, you are less likely to develop Alzheimer's compared to your risk if you had less education."

"Hmm . . . More education . . . ," John says, thinking. "What about if someone is smart but just never had the opportunity to go to college, would that also protect one against Alzheimer's disease?"

"Yes, absolutely. There are studies that support exactly that point—that being smart without a lot of formal education is also protective."

There are two main theories as to why higher education and intelligence may reduce the risk of Alzheimer's disease. The first theory is that education and intelligence enable you to build up a "cognitive reserve." The idea is that if the cognitive reserve is high enough then, for example, even if 25 percent of cognitive function is lost, there is still enough thinking and memory ability remaining "in reserve" for daily function to be normal. The second theory is that there is actually something different about the brains of people with higher education and intelligence and that brain difference makes it less likely that Alzheimer's disease will develop.

REDUCE YOUR RISK OF ALZHEIMER'S DISEASE BY AEROBIC EXERCISE, BEING SOCIALLY ACTIVE, AND EATING HEALTHY

"The other things that may be able to reduce your risk of Alzheimer's disease are doing aerobic exercise, staying socially active, and eating a healthy diet," explains the neuropsychologist. "Although there is a lot of active research going on right now trying to find out for sure whether these factors are truly protective, we are convinced enough by the studies that have already been published to strongly encourage all of our patients to exercise, be socially engaged, and eat a healthy diet."

Want to reduce your risk of developing Alzheimer's disease? There is increasing evidence that several lifestyle choices may help to keep your thinking and memory as strong as possible. We'll learn more about healthy eating and exercise in Step 5 and the importance of social activities in Step 6.

IN SPECIAL CIRCUMSTANCES A LUMBAR PUNCTURE CAN HELP TO CONFIRM ALZHEIMER'S DISEASE

"Is there a way to determine for sure whether the plaques and tangles of Alzheimer's that you were telling us about are in someone's brain?" asks Sue.

"In general, we make a diagnosis of Alzheimer's disease by doing just what we did in your evaluation," explains the neuropsychologist. "We listen to what the problems are, do pencil-and-paper tests, blood work, an MRI or CT scan of your brain, and a neurological evaluation. In certain situations that are unusual for one reason or another, we can do special tests that can detect the amyloid plaques in the brain. For example, if someone was, say, sixty-two years old and looked like he had Alzheimer's disease, we would recommend one of the special tests to confirm the diagnosis, as Alzheimer's disease is quite uncommon in a sixty-two-year-old."

"What are these special tests?" asks Sue.

"We can do a lumbar puncture—that's a spinal tap—and look for the levels of amyloid, which forms the plaques, and another protein called 'tau,' which forms the tangles. Certain changes in these levels suggest that the plaques and tangles of Alzheimer's disease are present in the brain."

Analyzing the levels of beta-amyloid and tau in the spinal fluid can help to confirm that Alzheimer's is present when the disease is strongly suspected but there is something unusual, such as the individual being younger than age sixty-five. Other things that may make the situation unusual would include early changes in movement or behavior. We don't use this test routinely both because it is not needed in the majority of individuals when the diagnosis is straightforward and because the test provides the right answer about 85 to 90 percent of the time but can be inconclusive or misleading the other 10 to 15 percent of the time.

A lumbar puncture—more commonly known as a spinal tap—may sound frightening, but it is actually a very safe and simple test that is less painful for most people than having an IV (intravenous line or catheter) placed. If your doctor suggests this test, you would begin by either sitting or lying down on your side with your back to the doctor and curling into a little ball by bringing your shoulders down and your knees up. The doctor would find the right spot, clean the area well, give you some numbing medicine (like in the dentist's office), insert a very thin needle, and take a small amount of spinal fluid out.

AMYLOID AND TAU PET SCANS CAN CONFIRM ALZHEIMER'S DISEASE BUT ARE NOT PAID FOR BY MEDICARE OR OTHER INSURANCE

"We could also do an amyloid or tau PET scan, which would show us if there are plaques or tangles in the brain," the neuropsychologist says.

"What's a PET scan?" John asks.

"A PET scan is like an 'inside-out' X-ray. With an X-ray, the radiation beams go from the transmitter, through your body, and collect on a film or X-ray detector. With an amyloid PET scan, the radiation built into a tiny molecule that is engineered to stick to amyloid plaques. The molecule is injected through an IV in your arm, and if there are any amyloid plaques in the brain, it will stick to them. The radiation of the molecule sticking to the plaques is then detected on the X-ray detector. With a tau PET scan the process is similar, except that the injected molecule is designed to stick to the tangles."

"Well, I would have the spinal tap if you told me I needed it, but I would prefer the PET scan," Sue states.

"In the future, we may be routinely ordering these amyloid and tau PET scans. However, right now, although the
scans are approved by the FDA—the U.S. Food and Drug
Administration—Medicare and insurance companies don't
pay for them.

"So how do people get them?" John asks.

"Currently people either pay several thousand dollars out of
their pocket or they get the scan as part of a clinical trial—a
research study to test out new ways to treat Alzheimer's
disease. So, because the PET scans are not paid for by insurance and we generally don't recommend lumbar punctures
unless it would change something about how we would
treat you, these special tests are not done routinely."

Amyloid and tau PET scans can correctly identify when the
plaques and tangles of Alzheimer's disease are present 90 to
95 percent of the time. Most often, however, the diagnosis of
Alzheimer's is clear and these scans are not needed. As with
the lumbar puncture, when circumstances are unusual, they
can be helpful. Currently amyloid and tau PET scans are
not paid for by Medicare or other health insurance; if that
changes, it is likely that these scans will be more widely used
in the future.

NEW BLOOD TESTS TO DIAGNOSE ALZHEIMER'S DISEASE ARE BEING DEVELOPED

At the time of this writing, several blood tests have been developed to assist in the diagnosis of Alzheimer's disease. It is our
opinion that none of the currently available blood tests are
sensitive or specific enough to reliably diagnose Alzheimer's
disease, and for that reason we do not recommend their use.
However, new blood tests are being developed every year, and
we are optimistic that within a few years there will be a blood

test good enough for us to recommend. We therefore suggest that if your doctor is concerned that you may have Alzheimer's, you ask them if they think a blood test to diagnose Alzheimer's disease could be helpful.

SUMMARY

"Maybe I should get one of these amyloid PET scans so I would know if I had the Alzheimer's plaques in my brain. Maybe I could enter a clinical trial . . ." Sue says, trailing off.

"You could definitely do that if you wanted to. But even if Alzheimer's disease were present, that wouldn't change the fact that we think it is very important to first address the issues of the sleeping medicine, alcohol, vitamins B$_{12}$ and D, and low thyroid. What about if we work together with your primary doctor to resolve these issues and have you come back in about three months to recheck your memory and see how it is doing at that point? My hope is that your thinking and memory will be noticeably clearer after those issues have been resolved."

"OK, that sounds like a good plan," Sue agrees.

Alzheimer's is a disease in which amyloid plaques build up in the brain. The plaques damage brain cells, the cells develop tangles, and the tangles destroy the cells. The Alzheimer's disease process begins asymptomatically and progresses through the mild cognitive impairment and very mild, mild, moderate, and severe dementia stages. Age, being a woman, family history, and head trauma are risk factors for the disease, whereas education, intelligence, aerobic exercise, social activities, and healthy eating may protect against developing it. Lastly, there are tests using a lumbar puncture or PET scan that can help to confirm the diagnosis of Alzheimer's disease, but they are only used in special circumstances.

Let's consider some examples to illustrate what we learned in this chapter.

- You've been told that you have mild cognitive impairment due to Alzheimer's disease. Does that mean that you have dementia?
  o No. There are different stages of Alzheimer's disease. The mild cognitive impairment stage means that there is difficulty with thinking and memory due to the plaques and tangles of Alzheimer's disease, but daily function is normal.
- Your friend told you that there is nothing you can do about Alzheimer's disease because if we live long enough everyone will get it. Is that true?
  o No. Alzheimer's disease is more common in aging, but many people live to age ninety or one hundred without the disease. Aerobic exercise, social activities, and healthy eating can all help reduce your chances of developing Alzheimer's disease.
- One of my parents developed Alzheimer's disease around age seventy-five. Does that mean that my chances of getting the disease are 50 percent?
  o No, although your chances are between two and four times more likely that you will develop Alzheimer's disease compared with someone without a family history of it.
- I'm having memory problems, but there is no history of Alzheimer's disease in my family. Does that mean there must be some other cause of my memory problems?
  o Although the risk is less without a family history, everyone is at risk for Alzheimer's disease as they get older.
- I'm worried about my memory, and I can afford to get one of those amyloid PET scans. Shouldn't I just have my doctor order one and not bother with the rest of the evaluation?
  o No. Even if the scan suggests Alzheimer's disease, there could still be other treatable factors impairing your memory that can only be identified during the regular evaluation.

9

What Are Vascular Dementia and Vascular Mild Cognitive Impairment?

After having learned about Alzheimer's disease in Chapter 8, we're ready to discuss other common disorders that can cause problems with thinking and memory. In this chapter we will learn that cerebrovascular disease (more commonly known as strokes) commonly contributes to cognitive impairment and is sometimes the sole cause of thinking and memory problems.

STROKES, ALSO CALLED VASCULAR OR CEREBROVASCULAR DISEASE, OCCUR WHEN A SMALL PART OF THE BRAIN DIES BECAUSE OF LACK OF BLOOD

We last saw Jack in his doctor's office. She had just told him that he had mild cognitive impairment because, although his day-to-day function is normal, his thinking and memory are mildly impaired. Let's catch up with Jack now as he and his daughter, Sara, are continuing their conversation with the doctor.

"So what's the cause of my 'mild cognitive impairment,' Doc?" Jack asks anxiously.

"I believe that there are actually two disorders that are each contributing to the mild problems you are experiencing in thinking and memory."

"TWO?!" Jack interjects. "You're telling me that I've got two disorders? What are they?"

"Dad, don't interrupt. She was just about to tell us," Sara says.

"I understand that this is a difficult conversation for you. I promise that I will explain everything and answer all of your questions—and you are free to interrupt me at any time," she says, punctuating her sentence with a little smile. "Now, in someone your age, seventy-two years old, the pattern of very mild memory problems that you are having is most likely caused by Alzheimer's disease. I think that is the first disorder."

She pauses while continuing to look at Jack. Jack nods, his jaw set. "OK, Doc," he says, "what's the other problem?"

"Your brain MRI scan shows that you have had some very small strokes, and I think that they are likely a contributing factor to your memory difficulties."

"What's a stroke?" asks Sara.

"A stroke is when blockage of one of the arteries, the vessels that carry blood from the heart to the brain, prevents a part of the brain from getting enough oxygen and other nutrients. The part of the brain that is blocked dies."

"What causes strokes?" asks Sara.

"Two main factors explain most strokes. The first is cholesterol building up on the inside of the arteries, which causes their openings to become narrow impeding the blood flow. The second is blood clots, which form either because the heart isn't pumping well or because the blood itself is too sticky. These clots can travel into the narrow arteries and plug them up."

Strokes occur when an artery sending blood from the heart to the brain becomes blocked off; that part of the brain doesn't receive enough blood and dies. Because the problem is related to blood vessels, strokes are often called "vascular disease" or sometimes "cerebrovascular disease" to emphasize the problem is with blood vessels of the brain or "cerebrum."

REDUCE YOUR RISK OF STROKE BY CONTROLLING MEDICAL AND LIFESTYLE FACTORS

"OK, so I think I understand what a stroke is," Sara says, "but why do people get them?"

"We understand some of the factors that lead people to develop strokes. They include any type of heart disease (including an abnormal heart rhythm or having had a heart attack), high blood pressure, high cholesterol, diabetes, smoking, lack of exercise, and—believe it or not—just being older."

"So I know I've got blood pressure and cholesterol, but you've got me taking pills for those," Jack says. "Are they still causing strokes if I'm taking pills?"

"Good question, and one that I want to talk about with you. The answer is that the risk of stroke is much less when these factors are treated, but the increased tendency toward strokes doesn't disappear entirely. In fact, because we now know that you have had these strokes, we are going to be more aggressive in treating your blood pressure and cholesterol and aim for a lower target for each."

"Is there anything else that my dad can do so that he doesn't have other strokes?" asks Sara.

"Staying active and exercising, keeping a healthy body weight, eating a healthy diet, and limiting alcohol will all help reduce the chances of having another stroke."

If you have any of the risk factors in the list below, you are at increased risk for stroke. The good thing is that, with the exception of age, you can take charge of your life and reduce your risk of stroke. Work with your doctor to make sure that your medical conditions are under good control. If you are smoking, quit today. Learn how to exercise for better health and to eat a healthy diet (Step 5). Work with your doctor to keep a healthy weight. Lastly, if you drink alcohol, drink in moderation (Step 3, Chapter 6; Step 5, Chapter 14).

Major Risk Factors for Stroke

Medical factors
o Prior stroke
o Prior stroke warning sign (transient ischemic attack, or TIA)
o Heart disease
o Disease of other blood vessels in the body
o Diabetes
o High cholesterol
o High blood pressure
Lifestyle factors
o Smoking
o Sedentary lifestyle
o Unhealthy diet
o Obesity
o Alcohol more than one drink per day
Uncontrollable factors
o Old age: after age fifty-five, the stroke risk doubles every decade

SMALL-VESSEL DISEASE STROKES ARE TYPICALLY SILENT

Jack thinks about his neighbor who had a stroke that left him paralyzed on one side and unable to talk. "How could I have had a stroke and not know it?"

"There are different types of strokes. Some strokes result from when a large artery is blocked off. These 'large-vessel strokes' typically cause a major problem that is often obvious, such as sudden weakness or numbness of an arm or a leg, sudden loss of vision, or sudden impairment of speech. There are also 'small-vessel disease strokes' that occur when tiny, microscopic arteries in the brain close off, causing a very tiny stroke. These very tiny strokes are typically silent, and in fact they usually don't cause a problem unless people have a lot of them."

Although individuals and family members usually notice major strokes from the blockage of large arteries right away, small-vessel disease strokes from the blockage of small and microscopic arteries in the brain are typically silent. A brain imaging study such as an MRI or CT scan is needed to see these tiny strokes. It is only when large numbers of these tiny strokes accumulate that they cause problems with thinking and memory.

VASCULAR DEMENTIA IS DEMENTIA DUE TO STROKE; VASCULAR MILD COGNITIVE IMPAIRMENT IS MILD COGNITIVE IMPAIRMENT DUE TO STROKE

"Is that when these small strokes cause memory troubles, when one has a lot of them?" asks Sara.

"Yes, exactly," the doctor replies. "Problems with thinking and memory will develop only if one has many small-vessel strokes, although a single large stroke can cause problems all by itself. If thinking and memory are impaired because of strokes—large or small—to the point that one's day-to-day function is impacted, we call it vascular dementia."

"But you told me I don't have dementia," Jack interjects.

"Yes. In your case, Jack, if I thought that all of your memory problems were due to strokes, I would call it 'vascular mild cognitive impairment,' to indicate that the vascular disease is causing mild cognitive impairment—mild problems with thinking and memory and normal day-to-day function."

As discussed in Step 3, Chapter 7, there are many different causes for the conditions "dementia" and "mild cognitive impairment." When strokes are the primary cause of thinking and memory problems, we use the term "vascular dementia" if day-to-day function is impaired and "vascular mild cognitive impairment" if day-to-day function is normal.

IT IS COMMON TO HAVE BOTH ALZHEIMER'S DISEASE AND SMALL STROKES IN THE BRAIN AFTER AGE SEVENTY

"OK, doc, I think I've got it," Jack says. "I've got this memory problem but I function OK, so we call it 'mild cognitive impairment,' and it is caused by both strokes and Alzheimer's."

"Yes, Jack, that's what I think is going on."

"Is it unusual to have memory problems from both strokes and Alzheimer's?" asks Sara.

"It's actually quite common to have both strokes and Alzheimer's disease. Most people in our society who are over age seventy have had at least a few of these small strokes. Usually these small, silent strokes are not enough by themselves to cause memory problems, but when someone has Alzheimer's disease in the brain as well, these small-vessel strokes can make the memory problems worse."

When strokes are the only cause of thinking and memory problems, there are usually clinically apparent large-vessel strokes affecting strength, sensation, balance, walking, speech, or vision in the weeks, months, or years preceding the memory disorder. When there is no history or suspicion of strokes and silent strokes are just found incidentally on the MRI or CT scan, the cause of the cognitive impairment is typically small-vessel strokes plus Alzheimer's disease or another disorder.

SUMMARY

Strokes, large and small, can damage the brain and cause problems with thinking and memory, leading to vascular mild cognitive impairment or vascular dementia. Large-vessel strokes are typically noticeable and cause sudden weakness or numbness of an arm or a leg, sudden loss of vision or impairment of speech, or sudden problems with balance or walking. Small strokes are common, silent, and often contribute to cognitive problems in those with Alzheimer's and other brain diseases. You can reduce your risk of strokes by controlling medical and lifestyle factors.

  Let's consider some examples to illustrate what we learned in this chapter.

- You've seen your MRI scan report, and it says that you have "scattered T2 hyperintensities consistent with microvascular ischemic disease." What does that mean?
  o That's a doctor's way of saying that there is something on the MRI scan that looks like small-vessel strokes.
- You've been told you have "mild cognitive impairment," and your CT scan report says that you have "mild to moderate small-vessel ischemic disease." Does that mean that you have "vascular mild cognitive impairment"?
  o Not necessarily. Although you could have vascular mild cognitive impairment as the sole cause of your memory difficulties,

you could also have another disorder plus the contribution of small-vessel mini-strokes.

- Is it really important to stop smoking, eat healthy, exercise, keep a healthy weight, and drink only in moderation?
  o Yes! Modifying your lifestyle in these positive ways will reduce your chances of having a stroke, improve and/or lessen the decline of your memory, and make you feel better.
- You've never experienced a stroke, yet your doctor says that you've had one and she can see it on the MRI scan. How can that be?
  o Many strokes—especially small ones—are "silent," meaning that they may not cause any noticeable symptoms.

10

What Else Could It Be?

What Are Other Brain Disorders of Aging Affecting Thinking and Memory?

After learning about two of the most common causes of memory loss, Alzheimer's and cerebrovascular disease, we will finish Step 3 by considering several other common brain diseases that can cause mild cognitive impairment and dementia, including Lewy body disease, frontotemporal dementia, primary progressive aphasia, normal pressure hydrocephalus, and several others. Rarer causes of dementia, including human immunodeficiency virus (HIV) disease, multiple sclerosis, progressive supranuclear palsy, and others, are described in the Glossary at the end of the book.

LEWY BODY DISEASE: FEATURES OF PARKINSON'S DISEASE, VISUAL HALLUCINATIONS, ACTING OUT DREAMS, PLUS IMPAIRED ATTENTION AND MEMORY

When we last saw Sue, she had been given the feedback from the doctors at the memory center that, working with her primary care physician, she needed to address a number of medical and lifestyle issues that could be impacting her thinking and memory. Three months have passed, and Sue has worked on all of these issues. She and her husband, John, have arrived early to her appointment and are in the waiting room with some of the other patients and their families.

"I'm sorry that I made us get here so early," Sue says. "I just didn't want to be late."

"I agree," John says. "You never know how the traffic will be. And I know you're anxious to see how your memory is doing now that you have worked on the issues that were brought up at the last visit."

Sue looks at John nervously and then looks away. She doesn't think her memory is any better. She cannot stop worrying that she might be developing Alzheimer's disease. She cannot stop the feelings of sadness, hopelessness, and anxiety as they wash over her again. She feels helpless.

"Don't worry," John says, seeing Sue's sadness and distress. "Whatever happens, we'll face it together."

"Thanks, John. You're so kind," Sue says, looking at John, as a tear wells in the corner of her eye. She wipes it away with the back of her hand. John takes her hand and squeezes it. She feels somewhat better, but she now finds herself wondering what would happen to their relationship if she develops Alzheimer's disease.

"Did you get some bad news?" asks the woman sitting next to her.

Sue turns and looks at the woman. She has white hair, kind eyes, and a tremor causing her hands to shake. "No," Sue responds, sighing, "But I am worried that I'm about to get some."

"Well, you just have to take things one day at a time," the woman instructs.

"Thanks," Sue says as she and the woman introduce themselves and their husbands to each other.

Sue notices that the tremor, which had disappeared when the woman was shaking hands, is back.

The woman sees Sue looking at her hands and says, "I see you've noticed my tremor."

Embarrassed, Sue quickly turns her gaze.

"That's OK. It's part of my disease. I've got Lewy body disease. My doctor says it's the same thing as dementia with Lewy bodies, only my function is OK, so I don't have dementia."

"Lewy body disease . . ." Sue says, trailing off. "I haven't heard of that."

"Not that many people have. It's a strange disease. For me, it started when I began to see an animal, like a dog, in my bedroom. I would wake my husband up and say, 'There's a dog in our bedroom!' But he would tell me that there wasn't anything there. Isn't that right, honey?"

"Yes, there was never a dog or anything else there," her husband confirms. "But you moved around in your sleep as if there was a dog—and it was chasing you!"

"Right—that is another part of the Lewy body disease," the woman explains. "I started acting my dreams out while I was sleeping. I began moving around in bed so much that my poor husband has to sleep in another bed just so he doesn't get 'black and blue' with all the moving and kicking that I do at night. And then the next thing that happened is that my hands began to shake. Not so bad, but—as you can see—noticeable."

"Does the shaking get in the way?" asks Sue.

"No, not too much. When I'm actually using my hands, the tremor quiets down. It mainly happens when my hands are doing nothing, and just resting. So that's Lewy body disease."

"Thanks, but I'm still confused about one thing: Why are you in a memory clinic?"

"Oh, right, I forgot to mention that! The disease also makes it difficult for me to pay attention and remember. A lot of stuff is much harder than it used to be, like paying the bills and balancing the checkbook."

Have you experienced a tremor in your hands that started on one side, shuffling steps when you walk, visual hallucinations of people or animals, or acting out your dreams? You could have Lewy body disease, a common disorder that can affect thinking and memory. We use the term "mild cognitive impairment with Lewy bodies" if function is normal, and "dementia with Lewy bodies" if function is impaired such that the label of dementia is appropriate. It is called Lewy body disease because under the microscope we find Lewy bodies in the brain. Lewy bodies, abnormal collections of protein that interferes with brain cell function, are also present in Parkinson's disease. The difference is that in Parkinson's disease, the Lewy bodies are only found in one part of the brain, causing the common features of Parkinson's disease: tremor, slow shuffling walking, slowness of movements, softness of voice, reduced size of letters in writing, and diminished facial expression. In these other Lewy body diseases, the Lewy bodies have spread throughout the brain, and, in addition to the features of Parkinson's disease, they often cause trouble with vision—including visual hallucinations—and acting out dreams at night. There may also be dramatic fluctuations in attention and alertness from one day to the next. Some people who have been living with Parkinson's disease for many years will later develop mild cognitive impairment or dementia. Because it started with Parkinson's disease, in these individuals it is sometimes called Parkinson's disease mild cognitive impairment and Parkinson's disease dementia.

Lewy body disease impairs the frontal lobe system, and so the trouble with thinking and memory will be related to difficulty paying attention when new memories are being formed and difficulty in retrieving memories. Because Lewy body disease does not damage the hippocampus, once memories are formed they should not be lost. However, we should note that it is not uncommon to have both Lewy body disease and Alzheimer's disease. These individuals have both the features of Lewy body disease and those of Alzheimer's disease (Step 2, Chapter 3, and Step 3, Chapter 8)— including damage to the hippocampus and rapid forgetting.

Common Features of Mild Cognitive Impairment with Lewy Bodies and Dementia with Lewy Bodies

Thinking and memory problems
- Poor attention
- Difficulty with complicated activities
- Difficulty forming and retrieving memories

Features of Parkinson's disease
- Tremor
- Slow, shuffling walking
- Slowness of movement
- Softness of voice
- Reduced size of letters in writing
- Diminished facial expression

Visual disturbances
- Visual hallucinations of people or animals
- Difficulty seeing

Fluctuations in attention and alertness
- There may be dramatic variation in abilities between one day and another.

Acting out dreams (not just talking in your sleep; see Step 5, Chapter 13)

FRONTOTEMPORAL DEMENTIA AFFECTS PERSONALITY, BEHAVIOR, AND COGNITION

"Everybody here has something going on," the woman contin-ues. "Let me introduce you to some of the others here in the waiting room." She introduces Sue and John to a man in his mid-fifties and his wife.

Sue notices that the man isn't showing much emotion. She also notes that she isn't able to make eye contact with him—even when she is looking directly into his eyes.

His wife explains. "He has frontotemporal dementia. It began with him not completing projects. For example, one day he started to mow the grass, took a break and came in for a snack, and then started to watch TV. I asked him if he was going to finish mowing the grass and he simply told me, 'No, I'm watching TV.' And so the lawnmower just sat there in the middle of the half-mowed yard. He really had no idea that he should have finished mowing the lawn. Eventually I had to ask one of the boys in the neighborhood to finish it up. That incident sticks in my mind as when I knew some-thing must be wrong, because the man I married wouldn't have behaved like that. The same types of problems were occurring at work. Projects were piling up on his desk, half completed. At work he was spending most of his time fooling around on his computer . . ." she says, trailing off, and then pausing before she continues. "This part is a bit embarrassing to say, but I know that it is just part of the disease. He began to watch a lot of pornography, both at work and at home. So when I was mentioning that he would be watching TV or on the computer, that was what he was spending most of his time doing. Not surprisingly, he lost his job."

Sue is feeling somewhat uncomfortable hearing this man's wife discuss such private information in front of him. But he does not seem to notice or care. He sits there with mild inter-est looking at them as if they are discussing something that does not concern him. "Was that when you took him to the doctor?" asks Sue.

"Shortly after that. It was when he had no interest in getting another job that I called his doctor. The doctor saw us and then referred us here."

"I can only imagine how difficult this situation is for you and for your family," Sue says.

"Yes, it has been difficult," she says, sighing. "And not only emotionally. The latest thing is that we have had to put locks—actual locks—on the refrigerator and the cupboards or he will come down at night and start eating all the food in the house. And it doesn't matter what it is—jar of mayonnaise, box of cake mix—if we leave it unlocked, he'll eat it."

Frontotemporal dementia usually looks different than Alzheimer's disease in a few ways. First, most people with frontotemporal dementia start to show symptoms between the ages of forty-five and sixty-five, although in about one-quarter of individuals the disease is first detected after age sixty-five. Second, the most prominent symptoms are changes in personality, behavior, and trouble performing complicated activities—all related to poor frontal lobe function. Friends and family members of individuals with frontotemporal dementia frequently describe them as behaving like "different people." They often show socially inappropriate behaviors, have poor manners, make impulsive decisions, and engage in careless actions. They frequently show little sympathy or empathy for others. Loss of interest, drive, and motivation to do anything is very common. Some individuals compulsively perform repetitive movements. Others show a marked change in food preferences (often preferring sweets), engage in binge eating, or excessive smoking or drinking alcohol. Individuals with frontotemporal dementia are unable to realize or understand that anything is wrong with their behavior; it is family or friends who bring the abnormal behavior to medical attention.

Changes in thinking and memory are related, not surprisingly, to the frontal lobes not working properly—making it difficult to pay attention when new memories are being formed and to retrieve memories. The frontal lobes are also involved in performing complicated activities, so doing things like using a new software program, preparing a gourmet meal, balancing the checkbook, and setting up a new electronic gadget become difficult.

Common Features of Frontotemporal Dementia

General features
- Three-quarters of individuals present between the ages of forty-five and sixty-five
- Prominent change in personality—individual often seems like a different person

Changes in behavior
- Socially inappropriate behavior, including inappropriate social remarks
- Loss of manners
- Impulsive, rash, or careless actions

Apathy or inertia
- Loss of interest, drive, or motivation
- Decreased initiation of activity
- Neglect of self-care

Loss of sympathy or empathy
- Diminished response to other people's needs or feelings
- Diminished social interest, interrelatedness, personal warmth, and social engagement

Perseverative, stereotyped, or compulsive/ritualistic behavior
- Simple repetitive movements
- Compulsive or ritualistic behaviors
- Repeating the same words

Abnormal eating behavior
- Altered food preferences
- Binge eating or increased use of alcohol or cigarettes

o Putting inedible objects in mouth

Thinking and memory problems

o Poor attention

o Difficulty with complicated activities

o Difficulty forming and retrieving memories

PRIMARY PROGRESSIVE APHASIA AFFECTS SPEECH AND LANGUAGE

"Let me introduce you to some others," the woman says to Sue.
"Here is a former teacher—like you."

"Nice to meet you," says Sue.

"It is a pleasure to meet you," says her husband.

They all shake hands, but the teacher doesn't say anything.

"She has what the doctor calls 'primary progressive aphasia,'"
her husband says. "It means that she has trouble talking."

"Oh," Sue responds, "that must be frustrating."

". . . Yes," the teacher says. ". . . I know . . . uh . . . but I can't get
it out. That's my sproblem."

"Are you able to write instead?" asks Sue.

". . . No, . . . it's worse . . . uh . . . harder . . . writing."

"But you can understand OK?" Sue asks.

". . . Yes, . . . I can understand . . . In fact . . . um . . . they don't
know that . . . that is . . . uh . . . that I ken . . . they thought
I couldn't hear them . . . and . . . you know . . ." She trails off.

"I think," her husband says, jumping in, "that she's explaining
how people often don't realize that she can understand
most things, and so they act as if she can't understand them,
saying things in front of her as if she couldn't hear or spoke
a different language."

"Oh, that's terrible," Sue says. No one says anything for a minute.
Sue is thinking that she, herself, is having difficulty coming
up with words. She says out loud, "Do you mind if I ask how
it started?"

". . . I teach . . . taught . . . eighth grade smath . . ."

"You taught eighth grade math??" Sue interjects, "I taught eighth grade English!"

Sue and the teacher share a smile. Sue then waits, conscious that she needs to give her time to speak.

"...I had sproblem...first...um...finding tings to say...words...finding words. . . . Terms . . . uh . . . smath terms . . . couldn't get them out. . . . Students noticed . . . some . . . uh . . . help, give me the word. . . . Then parents and teachers complain that I...um...had this sproblem and...uh...OK, now...um...I'm trying to say . . . principal said I can't . . . uh . . . can't teach," she finishes, with her eyes tearful.

Sue, both sympathetic and scared for herself, is also becoming tearful again.

"OK, you two," the woman jumps in. "Hold off on the water works. Let's try to keep a positive attitude here. Remember, 'one day at a time.'"

Sue gives her best attempt to smile, not sure if she has succeeded.

Have you experienced any difficulty finding words? We learned in Step 1, Chapter 2 that difficulty finding the names of people, places, and other proper nouns is common in normal aging. When there is trouble finding ordinary words or difficulty with other parts of speech and language, however, it could be a sign of a disorder of thinking and memory. Although speech and language problems are most often seen in common disorders of thinking and memory such as Alzheimer's disease and vascular dementia, there are some individuals who present first and foremost with speech and language problems. These individuals have primary progressive aphasia.

Primary progressive aphasia has three common variants. In one variant, the difficulty is mainly finding and pronouncing words, with comprehension and grammar being normal. In another variant there is difficulty naming objects, comprehending single words, and even understanding what objects are used for. In the last variant there is effortful, halting speech with errors, distortions, and impaired grammar; comprehension is normal for simple sentences but may be impaired for complicated ones.

Common Features of Primary Progressive Aphasia

General features
- Difficulty with language is the most prominent feature, particularly at the start of the disorder.
- Language problems impair daily living activities.

Logopenic (word-finding) variant
- There is difficulty retrieving single words in ordinary speech and when naming items.
- Pronunciation errors are common.
- Difficulty repeating phrases and sentences is common.
- Comprehension is normal.
- Use of grammar is normal.

Semantic (word-meaning) variant
- Naming objects is impaired.
- Comprehension is impaired—even of single words.
- Comprehension is often impaired for what some objects are—not just their names.
- Difficulty reading and writing is common.

Nonfluent/agrammatic variant
- Speech takes great effort and is halting, with speech errors and distortions.
- Grammar is impaired.
- Comprehension of complex sentences may be impaired.

POSTERIOR CORTICAL ATROPHY AFFECTS VISION FIRST AND MOST PROMINENTLY

Have you found yourself going to the eye doctor repeatedly because you're having trouble with your vision and each time the doctor says there's nothing wrong with your eyes? It could be due to a brain disorder. Although there are many brain disorders that can cause vision problems, in some individuals the cause is a form of dementia. When vision problems are the first and most prominent symptom in dementia, we use the term "posterior cortical atrophy" because it is the back or posterior part of the brain that is most affected.

NORMAL PRESSURE HYDROCEPHALUS IS CHARACTERIZED BY DIFFICULTY WALKING, URINARY URGENCY OR INCONTINENCE, AND POOR ATTENTION

Are you experiencing a slowing of your walking and a need to run to the bathroom to urinate? If so, it is certainly worth speaking with your doctor about whether you have normal pressure hydrocephalus, one of the few brain disorders of aging affecting thinking and memory that can be stopped. In normal pressure hydrocephalus there is an excess of fluid in the brain. Studies show that after treatment with a shunt (the tube that drains the excess fluid from the brain), the deterioration of thinking and memory is halted and there is improvement in the walking and urgent need to urinate.

Common thinking and memory problems that occur in normal pressure hydrocephalus include poor attention, being easily distracted, difficulty performing complicated tasks, loss of interest in activities, and slowness in thought and movement. The frontal lobe system is impaired, making it difficult to pay attention when new memories are being formed and to retrieve memories. Because normal pressure hydrocephalus does not damage the hippocampus, once memories are formed, they should not be lost.

Normal pressure hydrocephalus is an uncommon disorder, and there are a number of other disorders associated with aging that may cause problems with thinking and memory, walking, and urinary incontinence. But because normal pressure hydrocephalus can usually be successfully treated—stopping the decline in function—it is always worth considering.

Common Features of Normal Pressure Hydrocephalus

Thinking and memory problems
- Poor attention
- Being easily distracted
- Difficulty performing complicated tasks
- Loss of interest in activities
- Slow thinking
- Difficulty forming and retrieving memories

Walking difficulties
- Slow walking
- Short or little steps
- Slow, multistep turns
- Poor balance
- Tendency to fall backward

Urinary problems
- Urgent need to urinate
- Increased urinary frequency
- Urinary incontinence

TWO DISORDERS MAY MIMIC ALZHEIMER'S DISEASE: PRIMARY AGE-RELATED TAUOPATHY (PART) AND LIMBIC-PREDOMINANT AGE-RELATED TDP-43 ENCEPHALOPATHY (LATE)

Let's imagine the following situation. You see your doctor because you've been noticing memory problems. Your doctor sends you to a specialist who thinks you have the beginnings of Alzheimer's disease and, because of some unusual features, performs either an amyloid PET scan or a lumbar puncture to confirm the diagnosis. To everyone's surprise (and your relief) the tests come back negative. So you don't have Alzheimer's disease. But what do you have? The answer may be one of two common disorders that can mimic Alzheimer's disease.

Primary age-related tauopathy (PART) is a disorder that can mimic Alzheimer's disease in the mild cognitive impairment and mild dementia stages. It is common in individuals in their eighties and nineties. Under the microscope, there are no amyloid plaques but there are tangles. The tangles cause brain cells to die and that causes the problems with thinking and memory. When thinking and memory problems develop, it can initially be difficult to distinguish whether they are due to Alzheimer's disease or PART. Over time, however, in those with Alzheimer's the disease continues to progress to more severe dementia stages, whereas in those with PART the disorder stops at either the mild cognitive impairment or mild dementia stages.

Limbic-predominant age-related TDP-43 encephalopathy (LATE) is a disorder that can mimic Alzheimer's disease at any stage, from mild cognitive impairment to severe dementia. It is common in individuals in their eighties and nineties. Instead of plaques and tangles, a different abnormal protein known as "TDP-43" is found in the brain, which damages and then destroys brain cells. Because the TDP-43 first accumulates in the hippocampus and anterior temporal lobes, the first two symptoms are memory and word-finding problems—just like in Alzheimer's disease. Some doctors can look at the MRI or CT scan and make a good guess as to whether the individual has Alzheimer's or LATE, but the best way to be sure would be to obtain either a lumbar puncture, amyloid PET scan, or tau PET scan. Note, however, that the treatments for Alzheimer's disease and LATE are the same.

CEREBRAL AMYLOID ANGIOPATHY MAY CAUSE STROKES OR BLEEDS

In Step 3, Chapter 8 we discussed how beta-amyloid accumulates in Alzheimer's disease and forms plaques. In some patients with Alzheimer's, the beta-amyloid also accumulates in the walls of small blood vessels in the brain. When this happens, we use the term "cerebral amyloid angiopathy."

Cerebral amyloid angiopathy causes two problems. The first is that the accumulation of the amyloid can make blood vessels narrower, leading to small strokes (see Step 3, Chapter 9). The second is that the amyloid in the blood vessel walls makes the usually elastic vessels somewhat brittle and liable to rupture. When blood vessels rupture, it causes bleeding. Usually these brain bleeds are small and do not cause noticeable symptoms. Sometimes, however, these bleeds can be large and cause permanent brain damage or death. Cerebral amyloid angiopathy is common in older individuals with Alzheimer's disease (particularly if they are over age ninety), but it can be observed in those with Alzheimer's at any age. Bleeding related to cerebral amyloid angiopathy may occur with certain types of anti-amyloid treatments, as we will discuss in Step 4.

SUMMARY

In addition to Alzheimer's and cerebrovascular disease, other brain disorders of aging that affect thinking and memory include Lewy body disease, frontotemporal dementia, primary progressive aphasia, posterior cortical atrophy, and normal pressure hydrocephalus. Each produces characteristic changes in thinking, memory, language, behavior, and/or movement that allow you and your doctor to know when to consider them as possible causes of your memory difficulties. There are also some disorders that can mimic Alzheimer's disease such as PART and LATE. Lastly, when amyloid accumulates in the walls of blood vessels, it is known as cerebral amyloid angiopathy, which can lead to strokes and bleeds.

Let's consider some examples to illustrate what we learned in this chapter.

- First you were having some mild trouble with your memory, and now you have had several episodes of seeing a person or animal that isn't really there when you were waking up or falling asleep. Does this mean that you're going crazy?
  o Not at all. Seeing people or animals that are not really there may be a sign of Lewy body disease. Let your doctor know about these symptoms; there are medications that can help.
- You've been noticing trouble finding words for several months and now wonder if that means you have primary progressive aphasia.
  o Although it is possible that you have primary progressive aphasia, because word-finding difficulties occur so frequently it could be part of a more common disorder such as Alzheimer's disease or vascular cognitive impairment—or just normal aging.
- Your walking has become very slow, and you need to rush more to go to the bathroom to urinate. Should you speak with your doctor about whether you might have normal pressure hydrocephalus?
  o Yes. Normal pressure hydrocephalus is one of the most treatable disorders of aging affecting thinking and memory. The outcomes are better when detected and treated early, so make an appointment to see your doctor today.
- You've noticed that your husband, now age fifty-seven, is acting odd. Although a kind and considerate person all his life, he doesn't seem to care about your recent diagnosis of cancer. He is now spending more and more time by himself. You're worried that he is perhaps depressed, although he doesn't seem particularly sad. Most recently he stopped going to work—you're not sure if he was fired or just stopped going. What's going on?
  o If your loved one behaves in the way just described, make sure he or she sees their doctor. Frontotemporal dementia, a brain tumor, depression, or drug or alcohol abuse are just some of the possible causes.

With the conclusion of this chapter we have finished Step 3: Understand Your Memory Loss. You now understand what the term "dementia" means and how it differs from mild cognitive impairment and subjective cognitive decline. You've learned more about the most common causes of memory loss, Alzheimer's disease and cerebrovascular disease (strokes), as well as some less common disorders. You've also learned about the important problems that your doctor needs to consider and "rule out," such as vitamin deficiencies, chronic infections, brain tumors, sleep problems, and medication side effects. Now that you have a better understanding of what your memory loss may be due to, we're ready to improve your memory in Step 4: Treat Your Memory Loss.

Step 4

TREAT YOUR MEMORY LOSS

In Step 4 we will learn about some of the medical treatments for memory loss and the diseases that cause it, such as Alzheimer's. We will discuss both the treatments that are available today as well as those treatments being developed for the future. We will also discuss how to treat the symptoms of anxiety and depression that often accompany memory loss (or worrying about memory loss).

11

Which Medications Can Help Memory Loss and Alzheimer's Disease?

Now that we have considered the major causes of memory loss, we're ready to treat it. We will concentrate on the treatment of Alzheimer's disease but also mention when these treatments can help with other disorders that cause memory loss. We'll also discuss some of the new treatments for memory loss being developed now that may be available in the next few years. The bottom line is that there are good treatments available today, and there may be even better treatments tomorrow.

TREATMENTS FOR MEMORY LOSS CAN BE SYMPTOMATIC OR DISEASE MODIFYING

When we last saw Jack, his doctor had just told him that she thought he had mild cognitive impairment due to both Alzheimer's disease and cerebrovascular disease (strokes).

Let's listen in now as she explains to Jack and his daughter, Sara, how she is going to treat his memory loss.

"OK, Doc," Jack says. "Now I understand what's causing my memory loss. Is there anything that can be done about it?"

"Absolutely," says the doctor. "I'm going to start you on a medication to help improve your memory."

"That sounds great," Sara says. "Will it stop the Alzheimer's from progressing?"

"That's a very good question. There are two basic ways that medications can help Alzheimer's disease. The first is that the medication could slow down or actually stop the disease process in the brain. The second is that it can help thinking and memory, even if it doesn't do anything to the underlying brain disease."

"I'm not sure I'm with you, Doc . . . can you say that again?" Jack asks.

"Sure. Let's think about memory loss like a clock ticking down. Now if we had a medication that could actually stop the disease in its tracks, it would be as if the clock stopped."

"That would be great," Sara says.

"Yes," agrees the doctor, "that would be great. Unfortunately we don't have any medications that can do that."

Sara looks disappointed.

"Now, if we cannot completely stop the disease, the next thing to consider is whether we can slow it down—slow down that clock."

"Well, that would be good, Doc, but isn't there anything that could actually improve my memory?" Jack asks.

"Yes, absolutely, and that is the type of medication that I would like to prescribe. Medications that improve thinking and memory can 'turn back the clock' on your memory loss, but they don't change the speed at which the clock is ticking down. They are symptomatic—they help treat the symptoms. Thinking and memory are improved—that's the turning back of the clock—but because this medication doesn't alter the underlying Alzheimer's disease process, the speed the clock ticks down—the rate of the decline—is the same."

Imagine that you have a sinus infection. You have severe pain in your face, a headache, and a high fever. You see your doctor and she tells you to take ibuprofen—a pain reliever—for the pain, headache, and fever. She also prescribes an antibiotic to kill the bacteria that is causing the infection. The first type of treatment—the ibuprofen—is symptomatic because it treats the symptoms of the infection. The second type of treatment—the antibiotic—is disease modifying because it works to treat the underlying cause of the infection.

It is the same with treatments for Alzheimer's disease. Some treatments can help improve the symptoms of Alzheimer's disease—the problems with thinking and memory—by *improving* thinking and memory. Other treatments don't help with the symptoms, but address the underlying cause of Alzheimer's disease—the plaques and tangles (see Step 3, Chapter 8 for details). We will discuss both types of treatments.

CHOLINESTERASE INHIBITORS "TURN BACK THE CLOCK" ON MEMORY LOSS

"The medication that I am going to prescribe is called donepezil. You might have heard of it by its brand name, Aricept. Although it's approved for those with Alzheimer's disease dementia, in my experience it works quite well in those with mild cognitive impairment due to Alzheimer's disease."

"How does it work?" Sara asks.

"It works by stopping the breakdown of a chemical in the brain called acetylcholine."

"This medication will improve my memory?" asks Jack.

"Yes. Most people experience an improvement in their memory equivalent to 'turning back the clock' on their memory problems six to twelve months."

"You mean my memory will be like it was half a year or a year ago?" asks Jack.

"Yes, most likely. There are some people, perhaps a quarter, for whom it has a smaller effect or no effect. But most people see an improvement."

"How long will it work?" asks Sara.

"It typically works as long as one keeps taking it," explains the doctor. "But it is important to note that although it can 'turn back the clock,' it cannot stop the clock from ticking down."

"Because it is not disease modifying?" asks Sara.

"Yes, exactly. Your memory will still get worse over time," she says, looking at Jack, "because the medication cannot stop the Alzheimer's disease from progressing. But your thinking and memory will always be better on the medication than off of it."

"What happens if I stop taking it?" Jack asks.

"Your memory would decline in about two weeks the amount that it would normally decline in six to twelve months."

"I'll keep taking it then—I don't want that to happen!" Jack responds.

"What are the side effects?" Sara asks.

"Most people do fine on this medication without any side effects, but maybe one in ten people experience an upset stomach and have loss of appetite, nausea, loose stools, or rarely vomiting. About one in fifteen people will have vivid dreams at night—not necessarily nightmares, but whatever dreams they typically have can seem very real. Maybe one in thirty people will develop a runny nose, increased saliva, or muscle aches. And maybe one in a thousand people will experience a slowing of the heart rate."

"How will we know if Dad has a slowing of his heart?" asks Sara.

"He might feel lightheaded, like he might faint, or he could actually faint. If either of those symptoms happens, you should call the office or 911 right away. We'll take his pulse to get his heart rate now, and we will take it again when he's been on the medication for a while. We'll get an EKG as well, just to be safe. Any other questions about this medication?"

Jack shakes his head.

"OK, good. I'm starting you on 5 milligrams a day for one month followed by 10 milligrams after that. Starting slow will give your body a chance to get used to the medication and reduce the likelihood of side effects. I'd like to see you back in two to three months to see how you are doing on the medication. Call the office if you have any problems before that."

Donepezil (available as generic and as the brand, Aricept), rivastigmine (available as generic and as the brand, Exelon), and galantamine (generic only) are called "cholinesterase inhibitors" because they all work by inhibiting cholinesterase, the molecule that breaks down acetylcholine. Acetylcholine is a chemical in the brain important for thinking and memory. Alzheimer's disease, Lewy body disease, and cerebrovascular disease all cause a reduction of acetylcholine. By stopping the breakdown of acetylcholine, the cholinesterase inhibitors help to bring acetylcholine levels back to normal. In a very real sense, Alzheimer's and these other diseases disrupt the balance of chemicals in the brain, and cholinesterase inhibitors help to restore that balance, improving thinking and memory.

Although cholinesterase inhibitors are FDA approved for Alzheimer's and Lewy body disease in their dementia phases, we generally start them in the mild cognitive impairment stage of these disorders and in vascular mild cognitive impairment as well. Our thinking is simply that if you are going to "turn back the clock" by six to twelve months to improve your memory, it's best to do so when your cognitive function is as good as possible. Additionally, there is evidence that Alzheimer's disease dementia can be postponed for at least one year by using these medications.

These drugs are relatively well tolerated, with the major side effects being related to an upset stomach, sometimes leading to loss of appetite, nausea, and loose stools (Table 11.1). Slowing of the heart rate is a rare but serious side effect, and so if you are taking one of these medications and you feel lightheaded

Table 11.1 Approved Medications for the Treatment of Alzheimer's Disease

Medication	Usual Dose	Benefits	Common Side Effects	Mechanism	Comments
Donepezil (generic and Aricept)	5 mg once a day for 1 month, 10 mg once a day after that; can go up to 23 mg	Improved: memory attention mood behavior	Loss of appetite Nausea, vomiting Loose stools Vivid dreams Muscle aches Runny nose Increased saliva Slowing of heart rate	Symptomatic: inhibits cholinesterase	Generally well tolerated; also comes in oral dissolving tablet
Donepezil weekly patch (Adlarity)	5 mg/day for 1 month, 10 mg/day after that	Improved: memory attention mood behavior	Rash Vivid dreams Muscle aches Runny nose Increased saliva Slowing of heart rate Loss of appetite Nausea, vomiting Loose stools	Symptomatic: inhibits cholinesterase	Few stomach side effects; patch stays on for a week at a time; remove patch slowly

Medication	Dosing	Benefits	Side effects	Type	Notes
Galantamine immediate release (generic)	4 mg twice a day for 1 month, 8 mg twice a day after that; can go up to 12 mg twice a day	Improved: memory attention mood behavior	Loss of appetite, Nausea, vomiting, Loose stools, Vivid dreams, Muscle aches, Runny nose, Increased saliva, Slowing of heart rate	Symptomatic: inhibits cholinesterase	Can be taken just in the morning to reduce vivid dreams
Galantamine extended release (generic)	8 mg once a day for 1 month, 16 mg once a day after that; can go up to 24 mg	Improved: memory attention mood behavior	Loss of appetite, Nausea, vomiting, Loose stools, Vivid dreams, Muscle aches, Runny nose, Increased saliva, Slowing of heart rate	Symptomatic: inhibits cholinesterase	Generally well tolerated

(continued)

Table 11.1 Continued

Medication	Usual Dose	Benefits	Common Side Effects	Mechanism	Comments
Rivastigmine capsule (generic and Exelon)	1.5 mg twice a day for 1 month, 3 mg twice a day after that can go up to 6 mg twice a day	Improved: memory attention mood behavior	Loss of appetite Nausea, vomiting Loose stools Vivid dreams Muscle aches Runny nose Increased saliva Slowing of heart rate	Symptomatic: inhibits cholinesterase	Side effects less if taken with food
Rivastigmine daily patch (generic and Exelon)	4.6 mg/24h for 1 month, 9.5 mg/24h after that; can go up to 13.3 mg/24h	Improved: memory attention mood behavior	Rash Vivid dreams Muscle aches Runny nose Increased saliva Slowing of heart rate Loss of appetite Nausea, vomiting Loose stools	Symptomatic: inhibits cholinesterase	Generally well tolerated; few stomach side effects; remove patch slowly

| Memantine (generic) | 5 mg once a day up to 10 mg twice a day | Improved: attention alertness mood behavior | Confusion Drowsiness | Symptomatic: inhibits glutamate and stimulates dopamine | For individuals with moderate to severe dementia |
| Memantine extended release (Namenda XR) | 7 mg once a day up to 28 mg once a day | Improved: attention alertness mood behavior | Confusion Drowsiness | Symptomatic: inhibits glutamate and stimulates dopamine | For individuals with moderate to severe dementia |

or faint, you should let your doctor know right away or call 911 (in most regions of the United States) for emergency medical attention. If you do experience a side effect from one cholinesterase inhibitor (donepezil, for example) it may be that another (galantamine, for example) might work better for you. The rivastigmine patch has fewer stomach side effects because it isn't a pill but is somewhat cumbersome and generally requires another person to put it on and take it off daily.

Most people do very well with these medications and stay on them throughout their lives. Because they are symptomatic medications, cholinesterase inhibitors can turn back the clock on your memory loss by about six to twelve months, but they cannot stop the clock from ticking down. That means that the medication is most likely still working for you even if you have noticed your thinking and memory becoming worse over time. When the cholinesterase inhibitors are stopped, most people experience a decline of six to twelve months of function in about two weeks. So we recommend that if you had a good initial response, you continue taking this medication.

YOUR IMPRESSIONS, THOSE OF YOUR FAMILY, AND FOLLOW-UP TESTING CONFIRM THE MEDICATION IS WORKING

Two months later Jack and his daughter Sara are returning to meet with the doctor.

"Hi, Jack. How are things going with the donepezil? Have you noticed any improvements? Any side effects?"

"Pretty good, Doc," Jack responds. "I do think my memory is better—about like it was a year ago like you said. I can now keep track of my calendar better and not end up in the wrong place or in the right place but at the wrong time."

"I agree," Sara jumps in. "I can tell that Dad is having an easier
time keeping track of things."

"That's great to hear. Any side effects?"

"I did feel nauseous the first few days I started the medication,
and then again for a few days when I went up to the 10 mil-
ligram dose. But not anymore," Jack replies.

"That's very common. Any other side effects?"

"None that bother me, but those dreams! You weren't kid-
ding, Doc, when you told me that I might have vivid dreams.
They're wild."

"So the dreams are not bothering you?"

"Not at all . . . I can't wait to get into bed to see what I'll dream
up next."

"OK, I'm glad you're enjoying the dreams," the doctor says,
smiling.

There's a knock at the door.

"Come in."

The nurse steps into the exam room.

"Jack, I've asked my nurse to repeat that brief pencil-and-paper
test that you did with her before."

"No, not another test!" Jack exclaims.

"Come on, Dad, it won't be so bad," Sara says.

"It will help us to confirm that the medication is helping you,"
the doctor explains.

"OK . . . at least I think I might remember one of the animals
and one of the words from last time," Jack says to himself
out loud.

"Oh, we're going to use a different version of the test this
time, so the animals and words will be different," the nurse
explains. "We always use a different version when we repeat
the test within just a few months."

"Great," Jack groans.

Whenever we start a new medication, we want to be sure that
it is working. For medications whose goals are to improve
thinking and memory, we would always like three types of

information: your opinion of whether the medication is work-ing, the opinions of your family, and follow-up pencil-and-paper testing of your thinking and memory.

If it is clear that the medication is working, we simply con-tinue it at the present dose. If the medication doesn't seem to be working and there are no side effects, we may try a higher dose; for example, we may try 15 milligrams of donepezil. If the med-ication isn't working and there are some side effects, we may try a different cholinesterase inhibitor medication—for example, galantamine extended release or the rivastigmine patch.

MEMANTINE IS HELPFUL FOR THOSE WITH MODERATE OR SEVERE DEMENTIA

Jack goes off with the nurse for his pencil-and-paper testing.

"I've been doing some research on Alzheimer's disease, and I read about this other medication besides donepezil. I think it was called memantine. Should my dad be taking memantine, too?" Sara asks.

"I don't think so, at least not at this time," responds the doctor. "Memantine—also known by its brand name, Namenda—is helpful for those who are in the moderate to severe stage of Alzheimer's dementia. Memantine helps mainly with attention, alertness, and initiation—all things that become a problem later in the disease. It doesn't improve memory, so your father is unlikely to see any benefit from it."

"Would there be any harm in trying it?"

"Well, that's a good question. The major side effects are drowsi-ness and confusion, although . . ."

"Drowsiness and confusion!" Sara interjects. "I certainly don't want my father to have problems with those things."

"Only a small percentage of patients have trouble with them but, interestingly enough, the side effects are more common in patients with mild memory problems, like your father. That's why I don't start memantine in patients with mild disease."

"OK, I got it. It sounds like it's better to not start memantine now."

Memantine (available as generic and as the brand, Namenda) works by interacting with two chemicals in the brain. It partially inhibits the function of a chemical called glutamate, and it also helps the function of a different chemical called dopamine. These chemicals are not generally affected early in the course of Alzheimer's disease, but they are later on, in the moderate and severe dementia stages. That's one reason why we don't typically prescribe this medication for people with mild memory problems.

Most people in the moderate or severe dementia stage of Alzheimer's disease, vascular dementia, or dementia with Lewy bodies do well with memantine, although it has only been FDA approved in the United States for Alzheimer's disease. In Europe it is approved for use in vascular dementia, and in our experience it can be helpful in that disorder and in dementia with Lewy bodies as well.

Drowsiness and confusion are the most common side effects that we observe. Because many individuals with moderate to severe dementia already have periods of drowsiness and confusion, we generally want to hear the family tell us that there has been a noticeable improvement for us to continue the medication. The last thing we would want to do would be to prescribe a medication that is causing drowsiness or confusion!

ADUCANUMAB REMOVES AMYLOID FROM THE BRAIN BUT HAS SERIOUS SIDE EFFECTS AND MAY NOT LEAD TO IMPROVEMENT IN FUNCTION

There's a knock at the door.

"Come in."

"Twenty-six!" Jack says enthusiastically as he walks in smiling. "I went up three points, from twenty-three to twenty-six! I'm back in the normal range!"

"That's great, Dad," Sara says, smiling back.

"And that's just what we would expect," the doctor says. "Most people improve two to three points on that test when they take donepezil or a similar medication. OK, there are just two more things I'd like to go over today. On the day that I prescribed the donepezil, we discussed the different ways that medications for Alzheimer's disease work. I explained that some medications, like donepezil, are symptomatic, improving thinking and memory by turning back the clock on memory loss, and other medications are disease modifying and slow down the rate of decline—how fast the clock ticks down."

"But I thought there weren't any medications that could slow down Alzheimer's disease," Sara says.

"I think you're probably correct," the doctor agrees, "but there is one FDA-approved medication that was designed to slow down Alzheimer's disease. Its generic name is aducanumab, and its brand name is Aduhelm. It is a special antibody that removes the amyloid plaques from the brain."

"Aren't antibodies what fight infections, like from bacteria?" asks Sara.

"Yes, but these antibodies are made in a laboratory, and they're specifically designed to stick to the amyloid plaques. Once they stick to the plaques, the body's immune system comes in and removes the plaques just like bacteria are removed."

"That sounds amazing!" Jack exclaims. "So how do I get this drug?"

"Well, because this is a very special type of medication, we would send you to a neurologist. The neurologist would need to first make absolutely sure that you have Alzheimer's disease by performing a lumbar puncture or ordering an amyloid or tau PET scan. Then you would be given the medication in their clinic through an intravenous catheter monthly."

"Every month?" Jack asks.

"Yes, every month. And you'll be periodically monitored by MRI scans to make sure you don't develop brain swelling or brain bleeds."

"How often does brain swelling or bleeding occur?" Sara asks.

"Approximately 30 percent of people develop brain swelling and 10 percent of people develop brain bleeds. However, the bleeds are generally small and most of the time the swelling goes away and the medication can be resumed."

"Is it expensive?" Jack asks.

"It costs more than twenty-five-thousand dollars each year for these—"

"More than twenty-five-thousand dollars each year!" Jack interrupts.

"But it's covered by insurance, right?" Sara asks.

"Currently it is not paid for by Medicare (unless you're taking it as part of a research study) or any insurance company, although that could change in the future."

"OK, Doc, let me get this straight. You send me to a neurologist where I get a spinal tap or PET scan to confirm my Alzheimer's. I get the drug through an IV each month. They do MRI scans to see if I'm getting the brain swelling or bleeding. And it costs about half as much as I made each year when I was working as an electrician. But this will cure my Alzheimer's, right Doc?"

"Well, that's a good question. There were two large clinical trials held over eighteen months. In one trial there was improvement, equivalent to slowing down the clock for three months. But in the other trial there was worsening, equivalent to accelerating the clock for three months. So most experts feel that we don't really know if this medication works or not."

"Only three months? That's less than the effect of my donepezil," Jack says.

"If it isn't clear that it works, has all these serious side effects, and costs a fortune, why would anyone want to take it?" Sara asks.

"Few people do," the doctor replied. "But I did want to discuss it with you since it is an approved medication."

A new class of medications is being developed to slow down Alzheimer's disease by using an antibody made in a laboratory to remove the amyloid plaques from the brain. Although we don't recommend aducanumab (brand name Aduhelm), the only FDA approved amyloid-removing medication at the time of this writing, there are similar medications that may be approved by the FDA—and covered by Medicare and other insurance plans—within a few years.

How do you know if these amyloid-removing medications are right for you? First, you should have a diagnosis of either mild cognitive impairment due to Alzheimer's disease or mild dementia due to Alzheimer's disease. That means that despite having Alzheimer's disease, your function is either normal or you only have difficulty with complicated activities such as paying bills or grocery shopping. Because these medications slow down the decline but do not improve function in Alzheimer's disease, we do not recommend using them in individuals whose dementia has progressed beyond the mild stage (see Step 3, Chapters 7 and 8, for a description of dementia stages). Second, your Alzheimer's disease needs to be confirmed by either a lumbar puncture or an amyloid or tau PET scan, as described in Step 3, Chapter 8. Third, you need to be comfortable with the route and frequency of the administration of the medication. These medications are given either by an injection or by intravenous (IV) infusion, usually once a month. Some of these medications are taken forever, whereas others are taken only until the amyloid is cleared from the brain. Fourth, you need to be comfortable with the possible side effects. All of these types of medications have the potential to cause brain swelling and/or brain bleeding, although how common those side effects are differs between medications. You should discuss these and other possible side effects with your doctor. Fifth, you need to be comfortable with MRI scans, as it is how you will be monitored for some of these side effects.

In brief, although we don't recommend aducanumab (Aduhelm), we expect safer and more effective amyloid-removing medications to be available within a few years. If you are interested in one of these medications, we recommend that you make an appointment to see your doctor today. The sooner you start one of these medications, the sooner you can alter the course of your disease and maintain your current function for a longer time.

CLINICAL TRIALS PROVIDE ACCESS TO MEDICATIONS NOT YET APPROVED

"Are there any medications that actually do slow down Alzheimer's disease?" Sara asks.

"Not yet," the doctor replies. "But there are other medications being developed to try to do that. Because they are not yet approved, they are in clinical trials. That's what I want to go over with you now."

"What are 'clinical trials'?" asks Jack.

"To know whether a new medication is safe and does what it is designed to do, the new medication is given to a group of individuals who are compared to a similar group of individuals who are given a placebo—a fake pill that does nothing but looks like the real pill—instead of the medication. Both groups are closely monitored to see if the drug is working as well as for any side effects that may occur. That's a clinical trial."

"So, it is research?" Sara asks.

"Yes, exactly," the doctor confirms. "Clinical trials are one type of research."

"Would I be able to stay on the drug I'm already on?" Jack asks.

"Yes, absolutely, you would stay on the donepezil. It is important that any clinical trial you might participate in be in addition to the standard, approved therapy. In fact, most trials for Alzheimer's disease require you to be on donepezil or a similar medication."

"It sounds great," Jack says cautiously, "only, how much does it cost, Doc?"

"Actually, clinical trials don't cost you anything. All costs are paid for by the company that makes the drug."

"OK, you can sign me up!" Jack says. "Only, I'd like to be in the group that gets the medication, not the group that gets the placebo."

"I should have explained more clearly. In a clinical trial you don't get to choose whether you get the medication or placebo; it is randomly assigned."

"But what happens if I get the placebo?" Jack asks.

"Let me step back one minute. There are definitely pluses and minuses of doing clinical trials. On the plus side, you may have the opportunity to take a new medication before it is generally available. On the minus side you may get a placebo instead of the medication. And if you do get the medication, it may have side effects or it may not work or both—evaluating those things are some of the reasons that the medication is in clinical trials."

Jack looks at Sara, uncertain.

"What are some of the things that my dad would need to do in a clinical trial?" asks Sara.

"Each trial is a little different, but, in general, he would start by doing some pencil-and-paper testing . . ."

"More tests!" Jack interjects.

"Yes," says the doctor, smiling. "More tests. After that, there are some blood draws, EKGs of your heart, and then typically for these studies there are also one or more brain scans."

"Like another MRI?" Jack asks.

"Yes, exactly."

"How often would we need to come in for these things?" asks Sara.

"During the initial parts of the trial you might need to come in three or four times in a six- or seven-week period. Then things typically get spaced out to every month or every other month."

"How long do the clinical trials last?" Sara asks.

"Typically anywhere from six to twenty-four months. Every trial is a bit different."

The cholinesterase inhibitor medications to treat memory loss, such as donepezil, work, and we recommend and prescribe them. As discussed, they can turn back the clock on memory loss for six to twelve months. This reversal of symptoms is very important and improves quality of life for individuals with memory loss and their families. It is our goal, however, to provide opportunities to do even more for those who are interested. The ideal therapy for Alzheimer's disease would be not only to turn back the clock on memory loss but to slow down the decline as well. At the time of this writing, it is our opinion that no therapies have yet been proven to slow down the decline of Alzheimer's. Currently, the only way that one can have the possibility of receiving such a therapy is to participate in a clinical trial. It is for this reason that we recommend that all of our patients consider clinical trials.

Clinical trials are not for everyone. Few people want to return to the doctor's office for more visits, pencil-and-paper tests, blood draws, EKGs, and brain scans. Some people don't like the idea that they could get a placebo instead of the real medication. Other people are concerned about possible unknown side effects if they do get the real medication.

Most people, however, actually enjoy their participation in clinical trials. Clinical trials are one way to actively take charge of your disease and fight it directly. The additional visits are not onerous and can provide additional times to ask questions. People who participate in clinical trials actually end up with better health care than the average person, likely due to the frequent medical monitoring. Lastly, people who participate in clinical trials enjoy knowing that even if their participation doesn't end up helping them directly, they are contributing to scientific knowledge that can bring better treatments or even a possible cure for the next generation.

THE GOAL IS TO MAKE ALZHEIMER'S DISEASE SOMETHING TO MANAGE, NOT SOMETHING THAT WILL DEFINE YOUR LIFE

"Do you really think that there will be a cure for Alzheimer's disease?" Sara asks.

The doctor pauses, and then says, "I think the goal for a disease like Alzheimer's is to make it something that you can live with, something that you can manage, like having high blood pressure or diabetes. We're working to make Alzheimer's just another chronic disease, something that does not define your life."

"That would be great," Sara agrees. "What do you think, Dad? Should we find out more information about clinical trials?"

Jack thinks about himself and his memory problems. Then he thinks about Sara, with so much life ahead of her and his granddaughter, just starting out. "Absolutely," he responds.

Today, our proven treatments for Alzheimer's disease are symptomatic. They can turn the clock back on the disease for six to twelve months, but they cannot stop or slow down the underlying disease process. New treatments in clinical trials now might be able to slow down the damage caused by Alzheimer's disease, perhaps as much as fourfold. Untreated Alzheimer's disease lasts approximately six to fifteen years from the stage of mild cognitive impairment to severe dementia. If we can increase that range even twofold—making it twelve to thirty years—with disease-modifying therapies, we've turned Alzheimer's into a disease that can be managed like high blood pressure or diabetes, not something that needs to define your life.

SUMMARY

Alzheimer's disease and other causes of memory loss can be treated. Today, cholinesterase inhibitors (such as donepezil) can improve thinking and memory by turning back the clock on memory loss by six to twelve months. New medications, currently available only in clinical trials, have the potential to slow down the deterioration caused by Alzheimer's disease. Although a cure may be unrealistic, the goal is to make Alzheimer's something you can live with, like any other chronic disease.

Let's consider some examples to illustrate what we learned in this chapter.

- Your friend told you that medications to help memory loss like donepezil (brand name Aricept) only work for a short time, so it's better to wait until you really need them. Is that correct?
  o No. We recommend that people start on medication as soon as it is known that the memory loss is caused by Alzheimer's, Lewy body, or vascular disease. Cholinesterase inhibitors like donepezil can turn back the clock on memory loss for six to twelve months. Because these medications cannot stop the clock from ticking, they cannot stop people from getting worse over time, but the medications are still working to help their memory.
- You've been taking donepezil for two months and you're not sure if it is working. You're still experiencing memory problems. Your spouse, however, thinks you are a bit better, explaining that although you still forget things, it is less often—the way you were last year. Should you continue it?
  o Yes. It is difficult for all of us to look at ourselves objectively. Family members can provide an important viewpoint. It is also important to keep in mind that the approved medications for memory are not miracle drugs—they can reduce memory problems, but not eliminate them.
- You've been diagnosed with mild cognitive impairment due to Alzheimer's disease and have been taking donepezil (brand name

Aricept) for about a year. You're worried that you are getting worse. Should your doctor start memantine (brand name Namenda)?

o Memantine has been approved for people with moderate to severe dementia, and our experience is that those are the people who benefit from it. People with more mild symptoms tend not to be helped and often have side effects of drowsiness and confusion.

- You're considering participating in a clinical trial, but half the people get a placebo. Should you still do the trial even if you might end up in the placebo group?

  o Clinical trials are not for everyone. Part of participation is accepting that you may end up in the placebo group. Although clinical trials may help you personally, the best reason to participate is to contribute to research that may help others in the future.

- You are thinking about participating in a clinical trial that lasts twenty-four months, but you are worried about committing to something for so long. Once you start, do you have to keep going?

  o You can always stop participating in a clinical trial at any time for any reason. There is nothing wrong with giving it a try and stopping if you don't like it.

- You have read about a clinical trial that has two parts. In the first part, half the participants are on the new medication and half are on placebo. In the second part, everyone is on the new medication and no one is on placebo. How can everyone be on the new medication in the second part?

  o Many clinical trials are designed in two phases: a placebo-controlled phase and an open-label phase. In the open-label phase, everyone is on the real medication. If you are interested in such a clinical trial, you can find out more by speaking with the doctors and researchers who are conducting it.

- You have been diagnosed with mild cognitive impairment (or another memory disorder) and are interested in participating in a clinical trial, but none of your doctors know where they are done or how to get more information.

  o One place to get more information about clinical trials going on in your area is to contact Trial Match at the Alzheimer's

Association: https://trialmatch.alz.org/, email trialmatch@alz.org, or phone 800-272-3900.

o Another good source of information is the national Alzheimer's Disease Research Centers funded by the National Institute on Aging, part of the National Institutes of Health in the United States: https://www.nia.nih.gov/health/alzheimers-disease-research-centers

o You can also go to https://clinicaltrials.gov/ and type in appropriate keywords such as "mild cognitive impairment," "Alzheimer's disease," or "Lewy body."

12

I'm Feeling a Bit Anxious and Depressed by My Memory Loss or My Diagnosis

What Should I Do About These Feelings?

Few medical issues in our society today are more feared than memory problems and Alzheimer's disease. If you have been diagnosed with a memory disorder or have noticed memory problems, it is normal to feel worried, anxious, or sad. In this chapter we will discuss these feelings and how to manage them. We will learn that although these feelings are to be expected, there are many things that you can do to feel less sad and anxious.

ANXIETY IS COMMON WHEN ONE IS CONCERNED ABOUT MEMORY LOSS, ALZHEIMER'S DISEASE, DEMENTIA, AND THE FUTURE

Sue is still in the waiting room of the memory center, awaiting her follow-up visit. Over the last three months she has worked on the medical and lifestyle issues that could be impacting her thinking and memory. She is feeling quite anxious and becoming a little tearful. Her husband, John, sees her distress.

"What's wrong?" John asks Sue.

Sue tries to answer the question. Thoughts begin to fly through her head. *What's wrong?* Sue hears John's words, still echoing in her ears. *I'm feeling sick, that's what's wrong*, Sue thinks to herself. *I think I'm going to throw up. I feel so weak and tired . . . I think I'm going to faint.* She can feel her heart bumping against her chest. *Maybe it's just because I've had such trouble sleeping*, she thinks. John is still looking at her, patiently, waiting for her to answer. *What's wrong?* she repeats to herself again. *Doesn't he know what is wrong? Why is he asking me?* She's afraid to say it out loud, for that will just make it worse, more real.

"I'm just so worried that they're going to tell me I have Alzheimer's disease," Sue responds out loud, becoming tearful again.

You may find yourself feeling a little anxious about your memory loss. Or maybe you're absolutely terrified that you may be developing Alzheimer's disease. The first thing to understand is that these feelings of anxiety are common. Many people who are experiencing completely normal, age-related changes in thinking and memory often become anxious that the changes they have noticed are due to Alzheimer's.

Maybe your situation is a bit different. Perhaps you have just been given the diagnosis of mild cognitive impairment, Alzheimer's disease, or another disorder, and you're anxious about what the future will hold. We've discussed the medications that can help in Step 4, Chapter 11, and in Steps 5, 6, and 7 we will discuss how you can take charge of your life and improve your thinking and memory. Read on!

Anxiety can be a tricky thing. Believe it or not, you could have anxiety and not even realize it. Anxiety may affect up to three-quarters of those with memory loss. In addition to feelings of nervousness and worry, anxiety can cause many physical symptoms such as an increased heart rate, breathing rapidly, sweating, nausea, and even diarrhea. Understandably, many people suffer from anxiety but attribute their symptoms to medical problems. On the other hand, many of these symptoms could indicate a very serious medical problem, such as a heart attack. If you are having these symptoms, it is important to see your doctor to look for medical causes, such as heart disease. But if your doctor has "ruled out" all of the medical problems that could be causing your symptoms, it may be that you have anxiety.

Common Symptoms of Anxiety
- Feeling nervous, restless, or tense
- A sense of impending danger, panic, or doom
- Increased heart rate
- Breathing rapidly
- Sweating
- Trembling
- Feeling weak or tired
- Trouble concentrating
- Trouble thinking about other things
- Stomach or bowel problems
- Difficulty controlling anxious feelings
- Avoiding things that trigger the anxiety

FEELING SAD IS COMMON WHEN ONE IS CONCERNED ABOUT MEMORY LOSS

In addition to feeling anxious about memory loss, many people also feel sad. Even when the changes in memory are normal for age and not accompanied by a disorder, feeling sad or depressed about these changes is common. Feeling sad is especially likely when one receives the diagnosis of a memory disorder. Similar to other life changes—such as the death of a loved one, retirement, or leaving an old home—adjusting to a new diagnosis can be associated with feelings of sadness and grief, which are normal emotional reactions. These feelings of sadness are usually temporary and typically resolve on their own. On the other hand, if the sadness lasts for an extended period of time (two weeks or longer) and impairs functioning, we typically call it depression. Depression is not normal and is not to be expected just because one is older.

Common symptoms of depression include sleep difficulties, daytime fatigue, physical slowing, loss of interest in living, and hopelessness about the future in addition to feelings of sadness, worthlessness, and guilt. Depression can sometimes be difficult to differentiate from a memory disorder. We hope that the information provided in this book can help you to distinguish them, but a formal evaluation may be needed to know, for example, whether mild cognitive impairment has caused depression or it is the other way around.

Common Symptoms of Depression in Older Adults
- Feelings of sadness
- Feelings of worthlessness or guilt
- Fixating on past failures
- Being tearful
- Irritability or frustration, even over small matters
- Memory difficulties
- Trouble concentrating

- Sleep difficulties
- Daytime fatigue and lack of energy
- Changes in appetite
- Often wanting to stay at home
- Physical slowing
- Physical aches or pain
- Loss of interest in activities
- Loss of interest in sex
- Loss of interest in living
- Hopelessness about the future
- Frequent thoughts of death

ANXIETY AND DEPRESSION CAN INTERFERE WITH THINKING AND MEMORY

The neuropsychologist's assistant walks over to Sue in the waiting room and explains that they are going to do some pencil-and-paper testing. Sue takes a deep breath, gets up, gives John her "here-we-go" look, and follows the assistant down the hall.

"Please read the following words out loud and try to remember them," she instructs as she flips over an index card in front of Sue.

"Airplane," says Sue. *Airplane, airplane, airplane . . . I need to remember these words*, she thinks to herself. The assistant flips over the next word.

"Jam," Sue says. *Jam, Jam, Jam, and . . . airplane . . . come on, Sue, remember the words. . .*

"Football," Sue reads. *Football and Jam and what was the other one?*

"Table," Sue says. *I'm never going to remember all these words.*

"Attic." *How can anyone remember all these words?*

"Tiger." *I can't remember these words.*

"Fan." *I'm sure I have Alzheimer's disease.*

"Hand." *I have Alzheimer's disease and that's why I cannot remember the words.*

"Bottle." *My heart is pounding.*

"Picture." *I think I'm going to faint.*

The assistant puts away the cards and looks at Sue. "Would you like to take a break?"

"No," Sue responds. "Just give me a minute. I'd rather get it over with."

"OK, no problem. Just let me know when you're ready."

Sue takes a few deep breaths, tries to relax, and feels her heart starting to go back to normal. *I have to stop worrying,* she says to herself. Now that she is feeling less anxious, she is feeling fatigued and worn out, despite the fact that it is morning. She feels as if she has done three hours of testing instead of three minutes. *I'm feeling so tired,* she thinks to herself. The sadness is creeping in. It feels pointless to do the testing when it seems clear to her that she has Alzheimer's. *Come on, you've got to get through this,* she thinks. She sighs. The assistant is looking at her. "OK, I'm ready for the next one," Sue says.

She is given two different connect-the-dots tests and told to work as fast as she can. Sue puts her pencil on the first dot, finds the second dot, and draws a line. *This seems so difficult . . . did it seem difficult before? Am I getting worse already?* She looks for the third dot, finds it, and draws a line to it. Her hand seems to move slowly, as if she were moving underwater. *Three dots down, and twenty-two more to go,* she thinks, sighs again, and looks for the next dot.

Sue completes several more tests.

"Do you recall those words you read out loud?"

Sue thinks, *Now what were those words?* Her mind is blank. *Oh no, I can't think of any of them.* She feels her heart pounding against her chest. *Come on, Sue, what were those words?* It seems that the harder she tries to think of the words, the more her mind becomes blank. *I feel lightheaded.* She feels a trickle of sweat roll down her skin. *I can't think of any of them. . . . This proves I have Alzheimer's.* "I'm sorry," Sue says out loud. "I cannot remember any of them."

The assistant shows Sue more words on index cards, asking her if each word is one that she had read out loud earlier. *Jam*, Sue reads silently to herself. "Yes," she says out loud. *Turtle.* "No." *Moon.* "No." *Picture.* "Yes." The test continues. To Sue's surprise, she is easily able to tell which words were the ones she read out loud before, and which she had not. *At least I did OK on that test*, Sue thinks to herself.

Anxiety and depression—without any other disorder—can impair thinking and memory. We discussed briefly in Step 3, Chapter 6 that anxiety and depression disrupt attention and frontal lobe function, making it more difficult for memories to be stored and retrieved. When one is anxious, it is also difficult to focus on anything other than what is provoking the anxiety. In depression, actions may be slowed down, and tasks can seem more difficult than they are. The bottom line is that even when the brain is completely normal, anxiety and depression can interfere with thinking and memory.

ANXIETY AND DEPRESSION CAN MIMIC DEMENTIA

About ten minutes later Sue and John are seated comfortably in the neuropsychologist's office. The neurologist is there as well.

"So how did I do?" Sue asks nervously.

"We'll be going over the test results with you in just a minute, but first we'd like to review where we are now in your evaluation and the medical tests that have come back."

"Yes, of course," Sue replies.

"When we last saw you three months ago, we talked about reducing or stopping the over-the-counter medication for sleep, reducing your alcohol consumption to one drink per day, taking vitamins B$_{12}$ and D, and evaluating your thyroid. I have your primary doctor's notes in front of me, and I see that your B$_{12}$ and vitamin D levels are now normal, as is your thyroid function. How are you doing with the alcohol and sleeping medicine?"

"Those things are going pretty well," Sue responds. "I've stopped the sleeping medication. Although I still have some difficulty going to sleep or waking up in the night, it's not too bad. And John and I now have one glass of wine or cocktail in the evening, followed by sparkling water with a twist of lime. We don't miss that second drink."

"OK, great," the neuropsychologist responds. "So now I'd like to go over today's test results with you, but before I do, I wanted to ask how has your memory been doing over the last few months?"

Sue looks nervously over at John, and then back at the neuro-psychologist. "I think it is worse. I feel like I can't remember anything. I . . . I think I must have Alzheimer's disease," Sue says softly.

Instead of responding to Sue's statement, the neuropsycholo-gist asks, "How has your mood been lately?"

"My mood?" asks Sue.

"Yes, how have you been feeling?"

"OK, I guess." Sue responds, trying to show her best everything-is-OK face.

"Sue," John says, "I think we should be honest about how you are feeling. Frankly, I've been quite worried about Sue. I think she's depressed. As she mentioned, she's convinced that she has Alzheimer's and that thought terrifies her. She's become quite tearful."

Sue's eyes become red. She doesn't say anything.

The neuropsychologist looks directly at Sue and says, "I can-not say today whether or not you have Alzheimer's disease. What I can say is that your testing today is very consistent with someone who has anxiety or depression or both."

"Are you saying that having anxiety or depression can impair my thinking and memory?" Sue asks.

"That's exactly what I'm saying. If one is anxious or sad, it is
    hard to concentrate. And if you can't concentrate, it's hard
    to remember things. Feeling sad can also slow down our
    actions and make tasks seem more difficult."

Many older adults who are experiencing normal, age-related
changes in thinking and memory often become anxious
when they misattribute those normal changes to a disease like
Alzheimer's, which can then create a vicious cycle as the anxiety about memory worsens actual memory in daily life. The
term "pseudo-dementia" has even been used to describe an
individual who has depression severe enough to cause memory
loss that looks like dementia. If you are anxious or sad because
you have noticed mild memory problems or been given a
diagnosis of a memory disorder, it may be that your feelings
of anxiety or sadness are actually making your thinking and
memory worse.

EMOTIONAL CHANGES MAY BE DUE
TO BOTH PSYCHOLOGICAL AND
BIOLOGICAL FACTORS

They spend a few more minutes talking with Sue about her
    mood, explaining that they believe she has both depression
    and anxiety, and it is likely that these feelings are interfering
    with her thinking and memory.
"I never thought that worrying about my memory would actu-
    ally make it worse," Sue says. "But I just can't help it . . ." she
    breaks off, swallowing.
"We understand. One thing we know about depression and
    anxiety is that they can be caused either by our reaction to
    something that happens to us or by independent changes in
    the brain, and sometimes by both."
"What do you mean?" asks John.

"It is normal to feel sadness about something that happens such as the death of a loved one, and it is normal to feel anxiety when worrying about getting a serious disease. Those are external things that can happen to us. One can also be more likely to feel sad or anxious due to internal changes in the balance of chemicals in our brain."

"What would cause those changes in the brain chemicals?" asks Sue.

"Many brain diseases can do that, including cerebrovascular disease—strokes—and disorders of memory, such as Alzheimer's."

"Are you saying that Alzheimer's disease is causing changes in my mood as well as my memory?" asks Sue, again distressed.

"No. I'm just explaining that one of the reasons that it is difficult to stop depression and anxiety is that there are biological changes in the brain that go along with the changes in mood. Even if there are no brain diseases at all, the depression and anxiety *themselves* can cause changes in the brain's balance of chemicals. Once the chemicals get out of balance it can be difficult to get rid of depression and anxiety without an intervention."

Our emotions, including feelings like anxiety and depression, can affect how well our brain works, making certain aspects of remembering and thinking more difficult. The opposite is also true. Internal changes in our brain caused by memory disorders such as Alzheimer's disease can affect our emotions and behavior. Changes in mood and behavior can, of course, also be caused by external life events, such as retirement, a new diagnosis, or the death of a friend. Because changes in mood, anxiety, and behavior can be caused by external life events, internal changes in brain chemistry, or both, treatments work best when they address the underlying causes with talk therapy, medications, or both. When treated effectively, the impairment of thinking and memory caused by depression or anxiety can be reversed.

MEDICATIONS CAN RESTORE THE BALANCE OF CHEMICALS IN THE BRAIN, HELPING MOOD AND ANXIETY

"There are several things that we recommend to improve your mood and anxiety," the neurologist continues. "I'm going to discuss medications, and then our neuropsychologist will discuss some nonpharmacological treatments."

"How do the drugs work?" Sue asks. "I don't want something that will make me feel tired or make my memory worse."

"That's a good question, and trust me, giving you a medication that would make you tired or impair your memory would be the *last* thing that we would want to do. The type of medication that I recommend is in the Prozac family. We call them 'SSRIs,' which is short for selective serotonin reuptake inhibitors."

"Will they help restore the balance in my brain?" asks Sue.

"Yes, exactly. They will help restore the balance of your brain chemistry by raising the level of the chemical serotonin, which improves mood and anxiety."

"Is there a specific one that you recommend?" John asks.

"In my experience, sertraline, whose brand name is Zoloft, tends to work the best to treat depression and anxiety in older adults who may be experiencing memory loss as well."

Brain chemistry is frequently out of balance in depression and anxiety, whether because of a brain a disease or an external life event. For this reason, medications are often very helpful in treating these disorders. Although all medications can have side effects, the SSRI class—and sertraline (brand name, Zoloft) in particular—tends to work well at low doses with few side effects. Note that for depression or anxiety caused by an external event, such as the death of a loved one, we think about the medication as a ladder that can help someone "get out of the hole" of depression. Once they are recovered, they can often stop the medication, just as after someone climbs out of a hole they no longer need a ladder. For depression or anxiety caused by a brain disease, the medication is usually continued, because otherwise the chemical imbalance will often return.

TALK THERAPY CAN HELP IMPROVE MOOD AND ANXIETY

"I'd like to spend a few minutes talking about some of the other things you can do to help your mood," the neuropsychologist says. "The first thing I'd like to mention is talk therapy. It is important to explore some of the reasons that you are so afraid of Alzheimer's disease. Talking through these issues is important . . . otherwise we're just treating the symptoms of depression and anxiety without treating their underlying cause."

"OK," Sue says, "that makes sense."

"Good. We'll also use cognitive behavioral therapy techniques to discuss strategies for keeping your mood up and your anxiety down. That way when you begin to feel sad or anxious you'll have some methods to cope with those feelings."

"That would be great."

"There are some other things I'd like you to consider trying as well. There is evidence that aerobic exercise, meditation, and relaxation therapy can each help with depression and anxiety. Some of these activities may appeal to you more than others. I'd like you to try at least one of them."

"Wow, I never knew things like that could help with one's feelings," John exclaims.

"Yes, there are actually good studies supporting all of them, with the exercise studies showing the strongest evidence. The last thing I'd like you to consider is joining our Memory and Aging Group. It's designed for older adults who are interested in learning more about memory and how it changes as one gets older."

Sue looks uncertain. She asks, "Is it a support group?"

> "Not exactly; this group is more like a class than a support group. Each week we'll talk about different aspects of memory, what's normal and what's not, and also discuss ways to help improve your memory."
>
> Sue still looks uncertain.
>
> "Just give it some thought, and don't knock the support group aspect of it. It is extremely valuable to learn that other people are having many of the same issues you are. You can also discover how they have learned to cope with similar problems."
>
> Sue looks at the doctor, and then at John. "OK, all these things sound great," she says, with hope in her voice. She takes in a deep breath, lets it out slowly through her nose, and then produces the closest thing to a real smile she's had in a long time.

If you are worried about memory loss or sad about a particular diagnosis, talking about it in groups or one-on-one can help. Talk therapy can accomplish many goals, including providing coping strategies when one is feeling anxiety or sadness, dealing with the underlying cause of these feelings, as well as with existential issues such as death and the legacy we will leave behind after we are gone. In addition to more general approaches, specific therapies have been developed to treat anxiety and depression in individuals with memory loss. Because these therapies target emotions—which have a specialized memory system all their own—they can often be effective even if some forgetting of the content of the therapy sessions occurs.

AEROBIC EXERCISE, MEDITATION, AND RELAXATION THERAPY CAN HELP ANXIETY AND DEPRESSION

Feeling sad or anxious about your memory loss but not interested in medications or talking with anyone about it? Three things that you can do on your own to help improve your mood are aerobic exercise, meditation, and relaxation therapy. Each has been proven to improve mood and lessen anxiety in older adults. Exercise has the strongest evidence showing its effectiveness, but there are also studies supporting the use of mindfulness training (meditation being one example) and relaxation therapy. We'll be discussing exercise in more detail in Step 5, Chapter 15. You can find out more information about meditation and relaxation therapy from your doctor or the National Institutes of Health (see Further Reading).

SUPPORT GROUPS CAN BE VALUABLE IN HELPING MOOD AND ANXIETY AND PROVIDING PRACTICAL ADVICE

If you are feeling depressed because you are concerned about the changes you've noticed in your memory, chances are that you've been keeping your concerns to yourself. You may not want to burden your family and friends, or you may be worried about how they will react and treat you if you share your concerns with them. Support groups can provide a safe space for you to talk about your concerns and, in turn, help others with theirs.

Memory and aging groups deserve special mention. They are not traditional support groups. Led by teachers, they are groups for older adults who want to learn more about how memory changes with aging. These types of informational groups are becoming more common. Some hospitals and clinics offer them and many are being offered as part of adult education classes.

There are also more traditional support groups that focus on helping individuals with a specific diagnosis. So, if you have been given a diagnosis of Alzheimer's disease or depression or another condition, joining a support group that will allow you to talk with people who also have that diagnosis can be helpful.

Lastly, as you gain more experience and knowledge, you can help others in return.

DON'T FACE MEMORY PROBLEMS ALONE

We all need help and support when problems arise. Memory problems are difficult enough to deal with when we do have support and are much more difficult when we are facing them alone. Enlist your spouse, children, siblings, other family members, or friends to be your allies when you are dealing with issues of memory loss. Improved mood and less anxiety are just some of the benefits that involving others will yield.

SUMMARY

It is common to feel anxious about changes in your memory and to feel sad if you have been diagnosed with a memory disorder. It is important to deal with these emotions, as feeling anxious or sad can worsen—or actually cause—memory problems. Because anxiety and depression may be due both to psychological factors and changes in brain chemicals, treatments with medications and talk therapy can be effective and may be best in combination. Aerobic exercise, meditation, relaxation therapy, and support groups are also helpful in treating depression and anxiety caused by memory loss. Lastly, don't face memory problems alone—enlist family and friends to help. Treating anxiety and depression can improve your memory, daily function, and quality of life.

　　Let's consider some examples to illustrate what we learned in this chapter.

- You've been feeling depressed lately and you think it might be affecting your memory. Is this possible?
  o Depression can both be a reaction to memory loss and cause memory loss. If you are feeling depressed, it is important to talk

to your doctor. Treating your depression will likely improve your memory.

- Perhaps you're feeling anxious and can't seem to remember anything. How do you know if your memory loss is causing your anxiety or your anxiety is causing your memory loss?
  - o Sometimes it can be difficult to tell if anxiety or depression is causing memory loss or it is the other way around. To sort these symptoms out, we typically try treating one symptom—whichever we believe to be the underlying cause—and see if the other symptom goes away. So, if your anxiety is successfully treated and your memory returns to normal, then we presume that anxiety was the underlying cause. If you are no longer anxious but you are still experiencing memory loss, then we would be concerned that memory loss was the underlying cause and we would treat your memory.
- You've been feeling a bit anxious and sad. You are not interested in talk therapy or medication. Is there anything else you can do?
  - o Yes! Aerobic exercise, meditation, relaxation therapy, and support groups can all help. See details in this chapter for more information.

Step 5

MODIFY YOUR LIFESTYLE

In Step 4 we learned about how to treat your memory loss using medications, and we reviewed some of the new medications that are being developed. We also discussed what to do if you are feeling anxious or depressed about your memory loss. Our goal in Step 5 is to let you know about some of the changes you can make in your daily life that can help your memory, reduce your risk of developing a disorder of memory, and/or potentially slow down the decline of memory loss. We start by discussing the importance of sleep and what you can do to make sure that you achieve healthy, restful sleep each night. We then help you navigate the multiple and often conflicting claims about diet—what foods you should and shouldn't eat to help your memory. Last, we turn to exercise: how it can help your memory, and also what type and how much you should do. These important lifestyle changes are things that everyone can benefit from, even if one's memory is completely normal.

13

How Can Sleep Help My Memory?

You've probably heard that sleep is important for your health. But can sleep really help your memory? Is it true that not getting enough sleep can increase your risk of Alzheimer's disease? In this chapter we'll review how sleep and memory are related, sleep disorders that are common in aging, and the relationship between poor sleep and Alzheimer's.

IF YOU'RE TIRED, IT'S HARD TO PAY ATTENTION

Sue is still in the office speaking with the neuropsychologist and neurologist at the memory center.

"The last thing that we would like to discuss with you today is your sleep," the neuropsychologist says.

"My sleep?" Sue responds.

"Yes, sleep is very important for memory function, and when you met with us earlier you mentioned that you were having trouble sleeping three or four nights a week. One reason you need a good night's rest is so that you're not tired the next day. When you're tired, it's hard to pay attention, and if you cannot pay attention to things, you won't be able to remember them. In addition, it is mainly during sleep when our memories change from being temporary—lasting for a couple of weeks—to being more permanent and able to last for years. So getting a good night's sleep will help you to form strong memories and keep those memories for a lifetime."

In Steps 1 and 2 we discussed how your frontal lobes are important for paying attention to information as it is coming in from the senses so that it can be bound together and stored as a memory by the hippocampus. For the frontal lobes to do this important work, you need to be alert and well rested. Think about having breakfast with a friend. After a good night's sleep you can keep track and store memories such as what you ordered for breakfast (granola and yogurt with mixed berries), what your friend ordered (eggs sunny side up, bacon, and hash browns), the details of what your friend talked about (her granddaughter just started college and joined a sorority that is involved in charity work), what you told her about (that you've been reading a new book about the environment), and perhaps even the name of your waitress. Now imagine that your sleep the night before was disrupted and you're tired. Your tired frontal lobes will never be able to pay attention and keep track of all those details correctly. When you're tired, you might be able to take in the outlines of the memory—that you had breakfast with your friend—but not all the details.

SLEEP FACILITATES CONSOLIDATION OF MEMORIES

In Step 1, Chapter 1, we discussed how the hippocampus binds together the disparate parts of an episode of your life to form a memory. In Step 2, Chapter 4, we mentioned how sleep is essential for the brain's ability to transform memories so that they are not only stored temporarily in the hippocampus but also more permanently in the cortex, a process known as "consolidation." When consolidation occurs, the connections are strengthened between the brain regions related to the sights, sounds, smells, tastes, thoughts, and emotions of the memory episode. Although consolidation can take place while you are awake if you are resting, the direct linking together of the different components of a memory occurs mainly during sleep. Some sleep stages facilitate the long-lasting storage of the memory, whereas other sleep stages (particularly rapid-eye movement or REM sleep) facilitate interconnecting that memory with all your prior memories as well as your storehouse of facts and knowledge. Consolidation generally begins soon after an event, but the process may continue over many months or even years.

SLEEP DISORDERS ARE COMMON

"I'd like to ask you some additional questions about your sleep," the neurologist says. "Are you still having trouble sleeping three to four nights each week?"

"Yes," Sue responds.

"Do you have trouble falling asleep, staying asleep, or waking up too early?"

"Some nights I have trouble falling asleep, and other nights I go to sleep on time but then am up for a couple of hours in the middle of the night."

"Do you snore? Do you ever thrash about when you are sleeping or act out your dreams? Do you ever fall out of bed?"

"I don't think I snore or move around like that while I'm sleeping . . . do I, John?" Sue says, turning to John.

"Nope, no snoring, thrashing about, or falling out of bed," John confirms.

Sleep disorders are very common. They are sometimes caused by medication side effects or other medical disorders. If you suspect that you may have any of these disorders, make sure you discuss your sleep with your doctor. If these disorders disrupt your sleep, they will disrupt your memory.

Obstructive Sleep Apnea

If your bed partner—or someone sleeping in the next room—tells you that you snore loudly, or if you wake up in the night gasping for air, you may have obstructive sleep apnea. In addition to disrupting your sleep, this disorder reduces the oxygen in your blood, which can directly damage the hippocampus and also increase your risk of heart disease and strokes. It's important to see your doctor immediately if you suspect you have this problem. There are several good treatments available.

Restless Leg Syndrome

Do you find that it is hard to go to sleep because you experience unpleasant sensations in your feet or legs—feelings of crawling, creeping, pulling, throbbing, aching, itching, or electricity? If so, you may have restless leg syndrome. See your doctor if these sensations are keeping you up at night. Sometimes acetaminophen can help (see details later in this chapter).

Periodic Limb Movement Disorder

If your bed partner tells you that you are periodically kicking them in the night disrupting *their* sleep, you may have periodic limb movement disorder. It is a common side effect of many medications, including some antidepressants, antihistamines, and antipsychotics. In addition to disrupting your bed partner's sleep, this disorder disrupts some of the stages of your sleep as well. It's important to see your doctor, determine if you have this disorder, and treat it if you do. It may be as simple as adjusting one of your medications or adding a small dose of another.

REM Sleep Behavior Disorder

During REM sleep when your eyes are rapidly moving, the rest of your body from the neck down is normally motionless— paralyzed actually. Have you experienced the phenomena of waking up from a nightmare only to discover that you are unable to move for a second or two? If you have (we have), you'll know it feels longer than one or two seconds.

If your bed partner tells you that not only do you kick them in the night, but that you seem to be walking, running, fighting, wrestling, or doing other coordinated activities while you are sleeping, you may be acting out your dreams because you are not paralyzed during REM sleep. This is called REM sleep behavior disorder. If you don't have a bed partner, you might notice that your covers are all kicked out in the morning or you may fall out of bed. Although we want you to let your doctor know about this problem right away, you can see if you can treat it yourself with the over-the-counter drug, melatonin. Melatonin can often reduce—and sometimes eliminate—these abnormal movements. See the section on melatonin later in this chapter.

SLEEP THE RIGHT NUMBER OF HOURS FOR YOU

"OK," the neurologist continues, "so you have trouble both falling asleep and staying asleep. Let's briefly go over your sleep pattern. What time do you get up in the morning?"

"About eight o'clock," Sue responds.

"Do you take any naps during the day?"

"I might lie down and close my eyes for twenty minutes in the afternoon."

"And what time do you get into bed and try to fall asleep?"

"About ten o'clock."

"So that would be ten hours of sleep at night plus another twenty minutes from the nap," the neurologist calculates. "On average, people need between seven and eight hours of sleep at night, although some need a bit more—maybe nine hours—and others a bit less—maybe six hours. More than ten hours is probably more sleep than your body needs."

"But don't I need more sleep because I'm older?" Sue asks.

"No, that's a common myth. Somewhere between six to nine hours of sleep is the right amount for most older adults. My guess is that you are only having trouble falling asleep and staying asleep because you're trying to sleep more than your body needs."

"So what do you recommend? Should I cut out my nap?"

"It's up to you, but my recommendation would be to keep the twenty-minute nap but try either going to bed later or getting up earlier or both. Not everyone likes to nap, but those who do usually find a short ten-to-twenty-minute nap improves their memory and mental sharpness. Just make sure it's not too late in the day or it will be difficult to fall asleep at night."

"Why don't you try going to bed at eleven-thirty and getting up at seven like me?" John asks, jumping in.

Sue thinks about it, and then says, "So that would be going to bed one-and-a-half hours later and getting up one hour earlier, totaling about eight hours of sleep with the nap."

"That sounds like a good plan," agrees the neurologist.

Do you have trouble falling asleep, staying asleep, or waking up too early? One of the most common reasons that people have these sleep difficulties is simply that they are trying to sleep too many hours. Perhaps you used to go to bed at 10 PM and get up at 6 AM to get ready for work. Now that you're retired, however, you don't need to get up at 6 AM, so you set your alarm for 8 AM. Although sleeping from 10 PM to 8 AM may sound perfectly reasonable, it isn't, because you would be trying to sleep ten hours—too much for almost anyone! If your body did well with the eight hours sleep you had when you were working, trying to sleep ten hours each day would likely result in your spending two hours in bed each night when you are not sleeping, either trying to go to sleep, being up in the middle of the night, or waking up too early in the morning.

How much sleep is right for you? Most older adults need to sleep between six and nine hours each night. One way to determine how many hours of sleep you need is to think about how many hours of sleep you usually had when you were younger. If during that time of your life, you woke feeling well rested and were not falling asleep during the day, that is probably a good target to aim for.

Another way to calculate how much sleep you need is to add up the average amount of time you are actually sleeping in a twenty-four-hour period, including naps. Let's say you don't nap, you get into bed at 10 PM but don't fall asleep until 11 PM, are up for an hour in the middle of the night and, although you set your alarm for 8 AM, you generally wake at 7 AM, feeling rested. In this case you're waking up feeling well rested after seven hours of sleep. So seven hours is probably the right amount of sleep for you. This means that you would be unlikely to be awake in the middle of the night if you simply went to bed at 11:30 PM and set your alarm for 6:30 AM (or any seven-hour schedule).

NO PROBLEM WITH NAPPING

Naps are built into our biological clock, so there is nothing wrong with taking a nap. Most people who enjoy a nap find that their memory and alertness are better after taking a nap. Just remember that naps need to be included in your total sleep time. Naps should usually be ten to twenty minutes, never longer than one hour, and generally before 4 PM so that they don't interfere with your falling asleep at night.

MELATONIN AND ACETAMINOPHEN MAY HELP YOUR SLEEP

"I remember that you told me not to take over-the-counter sleeping pills because of the antihistamines in them," Sue begins, "but what about prescription sleeping pills? Are those any better for you?"

"Unfortunately not," the neurologist responds. "Most sleep experts believe that even the newer prescription sleeping pills don't produce normal, healthy sleep. The only two medications that we recommend for sleep are melatonin and acetaminophen."

Melatonin

Melatonin is a hormone that your body makes to help regulate your sleep cycle. When levels of melatonin rise, it tells your body to prepare for sleep. If you are having difficulty regulating your sleep cycle, you may benefit from taking melatonin, which is available over the counter. Let your doctor know if you are interested in this medication, however, as it can interact with other medicines. Start with a low dose, perhaps 0.5 mg, one hour before the time you wish to fall asleep. If a low dose is ineffective, you can increase the dose slowly as needed, but speak with your doctor if you would like to take more than 6 mg. *Never* take melatonin in the middle of the night or you may prevent yourself from falling sleep at a normal time.

Before you reach for that bottle, however, see if you can make your own melatonin by spending at least thirty minutes outside or near a bright, sunlit window between 1 and 3 PM. That sun exposure will help you to generate your own melatonin approximately eight hours later, between 9 and 11 PM.

Acetaminophen

Are you ever kept up at night by joint aches, back pains, sore muscles, or a stiff neck? Many people are. It is for this reason that acetaminophen (brand name Tylenol and many others), a mild pain reliever, can help you to fall asleep. But before you start taking acetaminophen, please check with your doctor. We recommend taking a single 325 mg pill about thirty minutes before your desired sleep time.

Sleeping Pills

What about over-the-counter sleeping pills like diphenhydramine (brand name Benadryl) and prescription sleeping pills like zolpidem (brand name Ambien) and suvorexant (brand name Belsomra)? Unfortunately, none of these pills produce natural sleep. Instead, they sedate you, and tend to impair your memory for events that happened earlier that day as well as for events you will experience the following day. Some studies have even suggested that prolonged use of sleeping pills is associated with an increased risk of Alzheimer's disease and others causes of dementia. Moreover, they only improve your speed of falling asleep by twenty-two minutes, on average. Twenty-two minutes is a small amount compared to their memory-impairing effects. We agree with the American College of Physicians who recommend not to take sleeping pills other than melatonin and acetaminophen.

DEVELOP GOOD SLEEP HABITS

"I'd like to also review your sleep habits," the neuropsychologist says. "Do you do any activities in bed, other than sleeping and sex?"

"Yes, I usually do the bills each month sitting in bed, that way I can spread them all out," Sue responds, adding, "Is that bad?" when she sees the neuropsychologist frown.

"The concern is that you're sending the wrong signals to your body about what the bed is for when you do an activity in bed that requires you to be wide awake, such as balancing your checkbook."

"That makes sense," Sue says. "I guess I could do the bills on the dining room table."

"Great," the neuropsychologist says, "that will definitely help your body feel more relaxed when you get into bed. Now tell me about any caffeinated beverages you drink, such as coffee, tea, and cola drinks."

"I generally have a cup of coffee in the morning, another one after lunch, and a third cup in the evening after dinner."

"My recommendation is to try turning that after-dinner coffee into decaffeinated coffee or herbal tea—and perhaps the afternoon one as well. Caffeine stays around a long time; after five hours only about half of it is metabolized—the other half is keeping you awake."

"Oh! I didn't realize that coffee could be keeping me awake hours later. I'll definitely switch to decaf in the afternoon and evening."

There are many habits and daily routines that can either be beneficial or detrimental to your sleep.

Tips to Sleep Better to Improve Your Memory

- Go to bed and wake up at the same time each day—weekends the same as weekdays. To find your ideal schedule, begin with a standard wake time. After a couple of weeks, you will find that you start to feel tired around the same time each night. Listen to your body and use that as your standard bedtime.
- If you nap, it should not be after 4 PM or for longer than an hour; brief ten-to-twenty-minute naps are best.
- It's normal for many people to spend fifteen to twenty minutes in bed before falling sleep; you shouldn't consider that a problem.

- During normal sleep there are several brief awakenings during the night; if you can return to sleep in ten to fifteen minutes (perhaps after using the toilet), this isn't a problem.
- Stimulate your own melatonin release by being exposed to sunlight first thing in the morning and for at least thirty minutes each day in the early afternoon (usually between 1 and 3 PM is best).
- Use a comfortable mattress and pillow.
- Bedrooms should be gadget-free (no beeps or lights), dark, and cool (generally between 65 and 68 degrees Fahrenheit).
- If you watch the clock trying to fall asleep or return to sleep, turn it around or remove it.
- Don't look at blue LED screens (such as on computers, tablets, and smartphones) prior to or in bed.
- Don't look at emails or do other nonrelaxing activities as you are going to bed.
- Reduce anxiety and worry before getting into bed. Read a book, listen to music, practice meditation, or take a hot bath. Try to establish a nightly routine that helps your body know it is time for sleep.
- Exercise during the day; this will help you fall asleep and sleep soundly at night. (Note: Exercise in the evenings or night can keep you awake.)
- Caffeinated beverages (such as coffee, tea, and colas) can keep you awake, so make sure you have them early in the day, perhaps just in the morning. Quantity matters as well. You may do best without any caffeinated beverages. Remember that "decaffeinated" coffee still has some caffeine it, as does chocolate.
- Don't use nicotine in cigarettes or in other forms. It is a stimulant and can keep you awake.
- Reduce your alcohol consumption, particularly in the evening and night. Although it may seem like alcohol helps sleep, it does not. Alcohol fragments sleep and causes many brief unremembered awakenings.
- Avoid large meals and beverages late at night. Fruit, although healthy, contains lots of water and may require your needing to use the toilet in the middle of the night.

- Some prescription medications that can be taken at any time of day will disrupt your sleep if you take them at night. Ask your doctor about whether some of your medications could be interfering with sleep. If so, ask if it is safe to move some of your nighttime medications to the afternoon or morning.
- If you have been lying in bed for thirty minutes and are getting anxious about falling asleep or are feeling activated—get up and do something quiet and relaxing in a different quiet and dimly lit room until you feel calmer.
- If you have been lying in bed for thirty minutes, and are not feeling anxious or activated, but are just relaxing and dozing, then you don't need to get out of bed. Dozing, relaxing, and daydreaming in bed with your eyes closed can have restorative value if it is during your usual sleeping time.
- If you're still having trouble falling asleep, try keeping a sleep log for at least two weeks. (Many activity trackers that are worn on your wrist can also help track your sleep.) Compare your log with the information you learned in this chapter. Track what time you get into bed, what time you try to fall asleep, what time you get up, how rested (or not) you feel, how many times you recall being up in the night (and for approximately how long), how many caffeinated beverages you consume during the day and at what time, how much exercise you do and at what times, the times and foods you have at your meals, and other information you think may be important. You'll likely see many ways you can improve your sleep.
- Lastly, it is completely normal to have trouble sleeping a couple of times each month. That isn't a sign that something is wrong or that you need to change your sleep habits.

SLEEPING THE RIGHT AMOUNT CAN REDUCE YOUR RISK OF ALZHEIMER'S DISEASE AND DEMENTIA

"Do you have any questions for us about your sleep and the changes you are going to make?" the neuropsychologist asks.

"Let's see," Sue begins. "I'm going to stay away from the over-the-counter sleeping pills I was using, sleep only eight hours each day—including my nap, do the bills on the dining room table instead of the bed, and drink decaf coffee in the afternoon and evening. All that makes sense. My only question is whether it's true that people who don't get enough sleep are more likely to develop Alzheimer's disease."

"Yes, studies have suggested that people who sleep less than six hours are at increased risk for Alzheimer's disease and other causes of dementia."

"OK," Sue says, "So that's another reason for me to try to sleep for eight hours each day."

"Absolutely," the neuropsychologist agrees. "We look forward to seeing you back in three months to see how your thinking and memory are doing after your mood, anxiety, and sleep are improved."

Many studies have found an increased risk of Alzheimer's disease and other forms of dementia in individuals who don't get enough sleep. One study found that individuals who slept five hours or less per night were twice as likely to develop dementia—and twice as likely to die—compared to those who slept six to eight hours per night. Another study found that sleeping less than six hours per night from age fifty to seventy was associated with a 30 percent increase in dementia risk compared to those who slept an average of seven hours.

Although no one knows for sure why inadequate sleep increases your dementia risk, it may be related to the beta-amyloid protein that forms plaques in Alzheimer's disease. It turns out that we all make some of this amyloid protein during the day. Normally, we flush away the amyloid while we sleep, a little bit at a time. So the idea is that if you don't spend enough time sleeping, you won't have enough time to flush all the amyloid out of your brain.

Lastly, inadequate sleep also increases your risk of weight gain, high blood pressure, diabetes, and heart disease—all of which increase your risk of strokes and vascular dementia.

SUMMARY

In this chapter we learned about the relationship between sleep, memory, and Alzheimer's disease, including that you need to get a good night's sleep both so that you can pay attention the next day and to facilitate the consolidation of your memories so that you can keep them for many years. We reviewed common sleep disorders and when to see your doctor if you suspect you have one of them. We listed a number of tips to sleep better to improve your memory, including making sure that you sleep the right number of hours, don't do wakeful activities in bed, and don't drink caffeinated beverages late in the day. We also discussed sleeping pills, and how we don't recommend them other than melatonin and acetaminophen. Lastly, we reviewed several studies that found that sleeping less than six hours could increase your risk for dementia.

Let's consider some examples to illustrate what we learned in this chapter.

- Your spouse says that you snore loudly and sometimes stop breathing when you're sleeping. But you've been doing that for years. Should you speak with your doctor about this long-standing issue?
  - o Yes! You may have obstructive sleep apnea which is treatable and—when untreated—is associated with memory impairment, heart disease, strokes, and death.
- You know that sleep is important for both memory and to reduce your risk of dementia. But the only way that you can fall asleep is with sleeping pills. What should you do?
  - o Speak with your doctor about cognitive behavioral therapy for insomnia. It works better than pills—and has no side effects.

- You understand that sleep is important, but you simply don't have time in your day to sleep for more than five hours. What should you do?
  - o Sleeping only five hours a day is like having untreated high blood pressure. You may get away with it for a time, but it will catch up with you and lead to poor health outcomes, including heart disease, strokes, diabetes, and dementia.
  - o Now is the right time to change your life for the better. Think about what changes you can make in your daily routine to allow yourself to sleep at least six hours each day.

14

What Foods Should I Eat or Avoid to Help My Memory?

Diet and nutrition are vital to maintaining cognitive health. Unfortunately, there are many different opinions out there about what you should and shouldn't eat for brain health. Making decisions about what type of diet to follow for brain health can be confusing. Should you drink red wine or stay away from alcohol? Are whole grains like quinoa and whole wheat good for you or do they cause dementia? Can you eat red meat or should you only eat poultry and fish? In this chapter we will review information about diet and the brain to enable you to make healthy dietary choices.

WHAT'S GOOD FOR THE BODY IS GOOD FOR THE BRAIN

Let's catch up with Jack and his daughter, Sara, as she is preparing a healthy dinner for them.

"I don't see that there is anything wrong with my diet!" Jack exclaims.

"Yes, Dad, I know," Sara says as she rinses the kale along with
red, yellow, and green peppers, "but I want to make sure that
we're doing everything that we can to help you with your
memory. I've been reading up and I've learned that there are
things that you should be eating to help your memory and
other things that can make your memory worse."

"You're saying that what I eat is important for my brain?"

"Yes, that's exactly what I'm saying."

The health of our brain is intimately related to the health of our
body. This statement is particularly true when it comes to the
health of our heart and our vascular system. We know that high
cholesterol, high blood pressure, and diabetes increase our risk
of stroke and dementia. The good news is that many of these risk
factors can be controlled through proper diet and nutrition. There
is no single "superfood" that has been shown to improve brain
health. Instead, the best advice is to eat a generally well-balanced
diet, consisting of many of those foods and food groups deemed
most beneficial for the brain and limiting those foods that have
been shown to be harmful when one has too much of them.

It's also important to maintain a healthy body weight in the
normal range for your height. Speak with your doctor or calculate your body mass index on your own using the National
Institutes of Health website (see Further Reading).

OMEGA-3 FATTY ACIDS MAY BE
HELPFUL, PARTICULARLY FROM FOODS

Sara arranges the kale and sliced peppers along with walnuts
and flaxseeds in a salad bowl.

"So what kind of lettuce is this?" asks Jack.

"It's not lettuce; it's kale," Sara answers.

"Kale? What's that?"

"It's actually a type of cabbage, and it is much healthier than
  lettuce, which has little nutritional value."
"OK, but why are we having nuts and seeds in a salad?"
"Because walnuts and flaxseeds, along with the kale, have omega-
  3 fatty acids, which is a type of fat that is good for your brain."

Omega-3 fatty acids (often shortened to "omega-3s") are important for a number of functions in the body, including the proper
function of our brain cells and reduction of inflammation.
Although our bodies make many of the fats we need, we cannot
make omega-3s, and so we need to get them from food. There
are three main types of omega-3s and, because you may have
heard claims about each of them, we'll mention them briefly
(despite their long names). Docosahexaenoic acid (DHA) has
been associated with brain health and cognitive function, control of inflammation, as well as heart health. Eicosapentaenoic
acid (EPA) has been associated with heart health and control of
inflammation. Alpha-linoleic acid (ALA) is a source of energy
and also a building block for both DHA and EPA. Scientific
studies examining the benefits of omega-3s have been mixed,
but some research suggests that they may benefit brain health.

Our recommendation is to make sure your balanced diet
does include some omega-3 fatty acids. The most common
sources of omega-3s include fish (particularly fatty fishes such
as salmon and tuna), walnuts, green leafy vegetables (such as
kale), flaxseeds, and flaxseed oil. Other foods are now being
fortified with omega-3s. You may find eggs, milk, juice, and
yogurt fortified with omega-3s in your local grocery store.

VITAMIN D IS IMPORTANT FOR BRAIN HEALTH

"So you're saying I have to eat the nuts, seeds, and all these
  vegetables?" asks Jack. "Can't I just take a pill?"

"Funny you should ask that, Dad. Although most nutrients are best from foods—especially vegetables—there are a few vitamins that are good to take in pill form. So I bought you two vitamin pills, vitamin D and a B-complex that includes B$_{12}$ and other B vitamins."

Vitamin D is essential for brain health. In one study, individuals with low levels of vitamin D were about twice as likely to develop dementia and Alzheimer's disease compared to those whose levels were normal. Most older adults don't have enough vitamin D. Although you can make vitamin D through your skin, to do so you would need to spend a lot of time outside without sunblock, which you shouldn't do. We recommend a daily intake of 2,000 IU of vitamin D$_3$, usually from supplement pills. You can also get vitamin D from fatty fish (such as tuna and salmon), portobello mushrooms grown under an ultraviolet light, and foods fortified with vitamin D, including milk, cereal, and orange juice. Be sure to read the label to see if the product you buy is fortified or not. Lastly, there are some important interactions between vitamin D and some prescription medications, so you should speak with your doctor prior to taking vitamin D supplements.

DEFICIENCY OF VITAMIN B$_{12}$ AND OTHER B VITAMINS CAN CAUSE MEMORY LOSS AND OTHER SERIOUS PROBLEMS

Deficiency of vitamin B$_{12}$ is serious, common, and easily treatable, so you'll want to make sure that your doctor checks you for it. Low levels of B$_{12}$ can cause numerous problems, including memory loss, hallucinations, fatigue, irritability, and depression, just to name a few. Some people, particularly vegetarians, don't get enough B$_{12}$ in their diet. Many older adults have difficulty absorbing B$_{12}$. If your levels are found to be low, the first thing to try is to increase your intake of B_{12} through vitamin B_{12} pills or by eating foods high in B_{12}. Liver and clams contain the most B_{12}, but fish and other shellfish, meats, milk, yogurt, and fortified foods also have some. If it turns out that you aren't getting enough B_{12} through intake alone, you may need to get B_{12} injections, which are generally given monthly until your levels are up to normal, and then less frequently after that.

In Step 3, Chapter 6 we discussed how deficiencies in vitamin B_1 (thiamine) can cause problems with thinking and memory. Links have also been shown between low levels of vitamin B_6 and Alzheimer's disease, leading people to wonder whether taking a B-complex supplement containing folic acid (folate), B_6, and B_{12} can help improve thinking and memory and prevent Alzheimer's disease in healthy individuals without any B vitamin deficiency. Studies have found little or no evidence to support the idea that taking a B-complex vitamin can improve thinking and memory or prevent Alzheimer's disease—unless one has a deficiency of these vitamins. We therefore do not recommend supplementation with B vitamins unless one has a deficiency, but neither do we discourage taking them. Your doctor can check to make sure that you don't have a deficiency of any of the B vitamins, and you can speak with your doctor about taking a B-complex or a multivitamin daily.

GET ANTIOXIDANTS FROM YOUR FOOD: EAT COLORFUL FRUITS AND VEGETABLES

Sara continues making the salad adding some little orange sections, fresh blueberries, and thin carrot slices.

"You're adding more vegetables?" asks Jack. "And what are those fruits doing in a salad, anyways?"

"The best way to get antioxidants, including vitamins A, C, and E, is by eating fruits and vegetables," responds Sara. "Just wait till you try it, Dad, I think you'll like it."

Antioxidants can defend the body against the harmful effects of free radicals—chemicals that can damage cells, including brain cells. Some of the most common antioxidants are vitamins A, C, and E, along with flavonoids and beta-carotene. Most studies looking at the impact of antioxidant supplementation through pills have offered little support that taking these antioxidant pills improves thinking and memory. In fact, taking high doses of antioxidants in pill form can be problematic, with some studies showing that high intake of antioxidants is associated with an increased risk of cancer and death. They can also negatively interact with certain medications. Thus, although some clinicians would recommend taking antioxidant supplements, such as vitamin E, we do not.

The evidence suggests that eating antioxidant-rich foods, such as fruits and vegetables, can reduce the risk of chronic health conditions such as heart disease and stroke, which, in turn, can improve the health of the brain. One study looked at over 75,000 people and found that those who ate more flavonoid-rich foods such as strawberries, oranges, grapefruits, apples, pears, celery, peppers, and bananas were less likely to show signs of cognitive decline as they aged. Many researchers now believe that it is the types and variety of antioxidant foods that people are consuming that matters most, rather than simply the total amount of antioxidants consumed. We therefore recommend eating colorful fruits and vegetables as part of a balanced diet.

MEDITERRANEAN-STYLE DIETS APPEAR TO BE MOST BENEFICIAL FOR BRAIN HEALTH

"So what meat are we having?" asks Jack.

"We're having fish," Sara says as she opens the oven door, dips a brush in olive oil and bastes a large piece of fish. Also

on the roasting pan are several garlic cloves and two large
onions. There are some avocado slices and lemon wedges
waiting for the fish on the serving platter.

"No meat? Not even chicken?"

"No. Fish, beans, and brown rice. I want you to see how delicious a healthy meal can be."

Jack inhales the aroma of the roasting fish. "Mmm . . . that
actually smells pretty good. Where did you learn to cook
like this?"

"I took a class on Italian cooking. These foods are all part of the
Mediterranean diet. It's one of very few diets that has been
proven to be good for your brain."

One of the most important ideas that has emerged from the
scientific literature is that it may not be any one dietary item
that makes a difference in the health of our brains. Instead, it
is likely that the complex combination of nutrients obtained
through a balanced diet is best. The Mediterranean diet (and
associated modifications such as the MIND diet) is one such
balanced diet that has shown promise for brain health. This diet
calls for high consumptions of fruit, whole grains (like bulgur,
barley, and brown rice), beans, and vegetables at every meal.
The diet is low in saturated fats (the "bad" fats) but encourages
the intake of monounsaturated "good" fats that lower the "bad"
cholesterol. These healthy fats, found in olive oil, avocados, and
nuts, should be eaten frequently. Fish is recommended at least
twice a week. Low to moderate amounts of dairy products such
as yogurt and cheese can be consumed daily or weekly. Red
meat and sweets (such as candy, cookies, cake, and ice cream)
should be consumed sparingly.

The Mediterranean Diet

- Fish
- Olive oil
- Avocado

- Fruit
- Vegetables
- Nuts
- Beans
- Whole grains (including bulgur, barley, and brown rice)

The MIND (Mediterranean-DASH [Dietary Approaches to Stop Hypertension] Intervention for Neurodegenerative Delay) Diet

- Olive oil daily
- Green leafy vegetables daily
- Other vegetables daily
- Whole grains daily
- Nuts and beans every other day
- Berries twice a week
- Poultry twice a week
- Fish once a week

One way the Mediterranean diet helps the brain is by reducing risk factors for stroke such as high cholesterol and diabetes. One study showed that brain volumes were larger for those who followed the Mediterranean diet, equivalent to being five years younger! Other studies have shown that people who eat a Mediterranean diet have a lower risk of subjective cognitive decline, mild cognitive impairment, and Alzheimer's disease dementia compared to those who ate a more typical diet. Several studies have shown that markers of Alzheimer's disease in the brain and spinal fluid (such as beta amyloid and tau) are lower in those who follow a Mediterranean diet compared to those who do not. Not all studies support the idea that the Mediterranean diet is good for cognition and reduced risk of memory loss, but most studies do, and none of the studies reported any side effects that would caution against adopting such a diet in an effort to keep the brain healthy. We therefore recommend a Mediterranean-type diet to everyone looking to improve their brain health.

Worried that some fish have high levels of mercury? Fish with low levels of mercury include Atlantic mackerel, black sea bass, catfish, clams, cod, crab, crawfish, flounder, haddock, lobster, salmon, sardines, scallops, shrimp, skate, sole, squid, tilapia, trout, and canned light tuna. You may want to eat swordfish and bigeye tuna only occasionally, as these fish have high levels of mercury. The U.S. Food and Drug Administration (FDA) has a good guide to help you know the levels of mercury in different types of fish (see Further Reading).

WHAT ABOUT RED WINE?

You may be wondering, "Hey, isn't red wine part of the Mediterranean diet?" You're correct, red wine has traditionally been part of the Mediterranean diet, and there are some studies that suggest one alcoholic beverage daily can reduce your risk of dementia. More recent studies, however, have questioned this finding. Many doctors and scientists now believe that the small correlations seen between moderate drinking and health are related to the fact that when people become ill, they generally stop drinking. In other words, it isn't that drinking keeps you healthy; it's just that unhealthy people don't drink.

Our reading of the literature is that a single alcoholic beverage neither helps nor harms your brain. However, as we discussed in Step 3, Chapter 6, even a single drink will impair your thinking and memory while the alcohol is in your body, and too much alcohol can increase your risk of cognitive decline and actually cause memory loss.

Our advice: If you enjoy a glass of wine with dinner, a beer at a ballgame, or a cocktail with friends, it is fine to continue to do so, limiting your intake to no more than two drinks per day and seven drinks per week. (Note, however, if you have any history of problem drinking you should not include alcohol in your diet.)

NO EVIDENCE FOR FISH OIL FOR BRAIN HEALTH

If fish is good for you, maybe you are wondering if you should be taking fish oil supplements. When it comes to supplementing your diet with fish oil, results have been mixed, and larger, more rigorous studies are needed to provide clear evidence of the effect of fish oil supplementation on memory. It also remains unclear what the appropriate dose of supplementation might be, with studies generally ranging from 180 to 2,000 mg and no clear indication of more benefit from higher doses. In short, if you are interested in taking fish oil as a supplement, we recommend you speak with your doctor. Nonetheless, we certainly encourage you to add one to three servings of fish to your weekly diet.

NO EVIDENCE FOR COCONUT OIL

There have been some claims that coconut oil may act as an alternative energy source to fuel the brain, thereby improving brain health, but no scientific studies to date provide evidence to support this claim. There are studies being conducted to explore this idea. There are currently no clinical data to support the idea that coconut oil may reduce risk of Alzheimer's disease and/or improve memory. We do not recommend taking coconut oil.

NO EVIDENCE FOR RESVERATROL, CURCUMIN, OR PREVAGEN

There are many supplements on the market today that are touted to reduce your risk of Alzheimer's disease and/or improve memory. Unfortunately, there is no evidence that any of them are helpful and therefore we do not recommend taking any supplements.

Resveratrol is found in red wine and blueberries and was thought be a protective factor against Alzheimer's. However, one carefully conducted year-long study found that giving people with Alzheimer's disease the amount of resveratrol in 186 bottles of wine each day made no difference.

Curcumin, one of the components in the curry spice turmeric, was believed to benefit thinking and memory. However, in our reading of the literature, there are no convincing studies that demonstrate any benefit.

The advertising for Prevagen boasts it is "the leading memory support and brain health supplement in America." Although we're sure it sells well, there is no evidence that this supplement containing a jellyfish protein works. In fact, the United States Federal Trade Commission charged its makers with false and deceptive advertising.

WE DO NOT RECOMMEND A KETOGENIC DIET

Two small studies, both with twenty or fewer subjects, suggested that the ketogenic diet could be helpful in people with Alzheimer's disease. However, larger studies are needed before we would recommend this high-fat, low-carbohydrate, adequate-protein diet. Although it can promote weight loss, its side effects include elevated cholesterol, constipation, kidney stones, and hypoglycemia (low blood sugar).

IT'S NEVER TOO LATE TO START EATING A HEALTHY DIET

"Dad, will you put the beans and rice into these serving bowls?"
While Jack is helping with the rice and beans, Sara takes the fish out of the oven and places it onto the serving platter. Together they bring the food to the table.

Jack takes a small bite of the roasted fish, beans, and brown
rice. "Hey, this stuff tastes pretty good," he says as he begins
taking some larger bites. To his surprise, he even likes the
salad with the kale, fruits, nuts, and seeds served with Sara's
olive oil and balsamic vinegar dressing.

"Sara, I really want to thank you for all that you are doing to try
to help me and my memory by showing me the right things
to eat. But I bet that I'm probably too old for a change of diet
to make much of a difference."

"You know, Dad, I was worried about that, too. But believe it
or not, I read that it isn't too late—even people your age and
older can change their diets and improve the health of their
brain."

"Really? OK. So, you're starting to convince me with all this
diet stuff. But what happens if I decide I want to eat a chili-
cheese corn dog or a Twinkie or fried dough once in a while.
Will all the positive benefits disappear?"

"I've got good news for you there, too. There's evidence that if
you can improve your diet most of the time, it will still help."

Are you interested in trying a new diet but wondering if you are
too old to benefit? Do you worry that the damage has already
been done from years of not eating properly? The good news
is that it is never too late to make a healthy lifestyle change
that will benefit your brain. One study found that older adults
aged fifty-five to eighty showed additional benefits of the
Mediterranean diet compared to eating a low-fat diet alone in
as little as four years.

YOU DON'T HAVE TO BE PERFECT

Let's face it—it's hard to be perfect. Most of us have tried a diet
before and found that it is hard to stick with it 100 percent of
the time. You may be wondering if there is any point in trying
to change your diet if you won't be able to follow the new diet

perfectly. A study investigating the impact of the MIND diet attempted to answer this very question. The researchers found that adults who followed the MIND diet "rigorously" had a 53 percent reduction in the risk of developing Alzheimer's disease. Importantly, even those nonperfect participants who followed the MIND diet "moderately well" were still able to lower their risk of developing Alzheimer's disease by 35 percent— quite a very large percentage! So you don't have to be perfect for a change in diet to help.

LIMIT CONSUMPTION OF BUTTER, MARGARINE, RED MEATS, FRIED FOODS, FAST FOODS, HIGHLY PROCESSED FOODS, PASTRIES, SWEETS, SODAS, AND JUICES

"Dad, I'm glad you brought up the chili-cheese corn dog and the fried dough, because there are some things that you should eat less of. Butter, margarine, red meats, cheeses, fried foods, fast foods, processed foods, pastries, sweets, sodas, and juices are all things that you should just have once in a while."

"OK, so you're not saying I can never eat chili-cheese corn dogs or fried dough, just that I shouldn't eat them every night," Jack says.

"Exactly! Anything you can do to improve your diet will help."

In addition to foods that can improve brain health, there are also foods that should be limited, including butter and stick margarine (less than a tablespoon a day), red meats, pastries and sweets, highly processed foods (like hot dogs), and fried or fast food (less than a serving a week). Try to reduce your consumption of these foods; even small changes can have a big benefit.

Note that you should also limit your consumption of sodas and juices, including those with artificial sweeteners. The problem is that both sugar and artificial sweeteners cause a spike of insulin in your body. This insulin spike is not good for your brain. It also makes you hungry and you end up eating more than if you drank water without the sweetener. Probably for these reasons, people who drink large amounts of sodas or juice—whether with sugar or artificial sweeteners—are at increased risk for developing cognitive impairment.

CHOCOLATE, IN SMALL AMOUNTS, CAN BENEFIT THINKING, MEMORY, AND MOOD

Sara and Jack clear the dinner and salad plates, along with the fish platter and serving bowls.

"Have a seat, Dad. I'll get the dessert."

"You mean I actually get dessert with this brain diet?"

"Yes," Sara says with a smile as she brings in some chocolate on a plate. "Chocolate is good for your thinking, memory, and even your mood."

"It tastes a bit strong," Jack says as he eats some chocolate.

"That's because it is dark chocolate. It is the actual cocoa that makes it healthy—not the sugar, fat, and milk added to the chocolate to make it sweet and creamy."

Jack and Sara continue to eat the dark chocolate.

"So if chocolate is good for you, what about chocolate cake?" asks Jack, hopefully.

"What I've learned is that although whole grains—like the brown rice we had tonight—are not bad for you, refined grains such as white flour, white bread, most pastas, donuts—and cakes—can be harmful. The problem with refined flour is that our bodies digest it very quickly and turn it into sugars,

> and so it can be just like eating lots of pure sugar. Chocolate cake would be OK to eat once in a while, but between the butter and sugar of the frosting and the refined flour of the cake it wouldn't be the right thing to eat frequently."

Good news for those with a sweet tooth! Chocolate has been shown to improve thinking, memory, and mood, and is also a source of antioxidants. The benefit comes from the actual raw cocoa, so the darker the chocolate the better. In the United States dark chocolate needs to have a minimum of 35 percent cocoa, sweet chocolate a minimum of 15 percent, and milk chocolate a minimum of 10 percent. (White chocolate has no cocoa in it.) You'll find that some dark chocolates, particularly those from Europe, advertise the percentage of cocoa on the package, with some ranging from 60 to 90 percent! The recommended daily dose of chocolate generally ranges from 0.35 to 1.6 ounces. So, if a typical chocolate bar weighs 3.5 ounces, the recommended daily serving size is about one-third of a bar. Be careful about overdoing it. Chocolate is high in calories, fat, and sugar, too much of which can be detrimental to thinking and memory.

EATING WHOLE GRAINS IN MODERATION IS NOT HARMFUL

Some people do think that eating any grains—even whole grains—is bad for the brain. This idea comes from connections between the intake of refined grains (such as white flour) causing blood sugar to rise rapidly, and gluten, which can cause inflammation in people with celiac disease (who are allergic to gluten). When grains are refined, the bran and germ are removed from the grain and there are many losses in nutritional value and fiber. The white rice or white flour that remains is almost pure carbohydrate—complex sugars that can be very quickly turned into simple sugars by the body. When these simple sugars are absorbed, they cause a spike in blood sugar that, as we mentioned, is not good for the brain. Thus, white rice, white bread, many cold cereals, many cakes and pastries, and most pastas are not good for the brain.

On the other hand, whole grains and things made from them, such as wheat and rye bread, oats, barley, brown rice, and quinoa, are nutrient rich, are converted to sugar slowly, and do not cause the same detrimental spikes in blood sugar. In addition, gluten is only associated with declines in thinking and memory for those who have a very specific gluten allergy (called celiac disease). Diets that contain whole grains (such as the Mediterranean-style diets we have been discussing) have consistently been linked to brain health. There is no evidence that moderate consumption of whole grains leads to an increased risk of memory loss and dementia for the majority of adults— unless they have celiac or a similar disease. The bottom line is that we do not recommend a grain-free diet. As discussed earlier, we recommend moderate consumption of whole grains and limited intake of refined grains.

SUMMARY

"All right, you've convinced me," Jack responds, smiling. "Any diet that lets me sit down and watch a ball game with a beer and a bag of peanuts doesn't sound that bad—and I can even have some chocolate for dessert!"

In this chapter we discovered how diet can impact brain health. We learned that there is no single food item that can improve memory, but rather it is important to focus on overall dietary health and maintaining a healthy weight. Mediterranean-style diets that emphasize increased consumption of fish, vegetables, fruits, nuts, beans, whole grains, and healthy sources of fat appear to be most beneficial to brain health. It is okay if our eating habits are not perfect, as long as we are generally consuming healthy foods. Importantly, it is never too late to start eating a healthy diet and reap the benefits!

Let's consider some examples to illustrate what we learned in this chapter.

- Your neighbor just told you that she has been taking omega-3 fatty acids and vitamin E supplements to protect her brain. You've heard that these nutrients are good for the brain, and you wonder if you should be adding supplements to your diet.
  - o Although some dietary supplements like omega-3s and anti-oxidants (such as vitamin E) have been linked to brain health, most studies have been mixed. It is more beneficial to focus on consuming a balanced diet that provides a variety of nutrients that work together—including omega-3s and antioxidants from foods—to help maintain the health of our brain.
- You keep reading about the benefits of a healthy diet, but have no idea where to begin. There are so many diet fads out there. Which is the right one?
  - o Mediterranean-style diets have the best, most consistent evidence of being beneficial for brain health. These diets emphasize high consumption of fruits, vegetables, whole grains, beans, and nuts. They are low in saturated fat and high in monounsaturated fat. Consumption of fish is emphasized, with low to moderate dairy consumption. Red meats and sugar are consumed sparingly.
- Your cousin has celiac disease and has stopped eating grains. She tells you that she feels much better and cognitively sharper. You've heard that eating grains can be bad for the brain and may cause dementia. Should you stop eating grains?
  - o There are certain conditions, such as celiac disease, that cause sensitivity to the gluten found in most grains. People with this type of specific allergy can experience changes in mental alertness and decline in memory when they consume grains. However, most people do not have this specific type of allergy, and so eating whole grains does not cause any problems with

thinking and memory for most people. There is no evidence to support the theory that eating moderate amounts of whole grains causes dementia.

- You know that you are supposed to eat a healthy diet and avoid certain foods like those that are high in saturated fat and sugar, but sometimes you just get a craving for a treat that does not fit with your healthy diet. You wonder if you should just give up on the diet entirely. If you can't maintain a healthy diet all the time, maybe you just shouldn't bother trying at all, right?

  o Wrong! Luckily, the research has shown that as long as we eat a healthy diet most of the time, our brains can still benefit. We don't need to be perfect; we just need to make sure we are generally trying to follow the dietary recommendations that benefit brain health.

15

Can Physical Activity and Exercise Help My Memory?

We all know exercise is good for us. We hear it from our doctors, the news media, and the talk shows. What's often not understood, however, is just how good exercise is for you and why. Not only does it help your heart, muscles, and bones, exercise is also critically important for your brain, too—improving your thinking, memory, and emotional health.

IT'S NEVER TOO LATE TO START EXERCISING

Let's join Sue as she is speaking with her doctor about exercise.

"When I met with the neuropsychologist," Sue begins, "she stressed that exercise was one of the most important things that I could do to improve my mood, reduce anxiety, help my sleep, and keep my memory strong. But as I was driving home with John from the appointment, I realized that I don't really know what I am supposed to be doing. I know it's supposed to be 'aerobic,' but I don't know exactly what that means. I'm also not sure what is the best type of exercise to do, how much of it I should be doing, and what is safe to do at my age of eighty.

I confess I have never been one to exercise. I also wonder if I'm too old to start."

"Those are all great questions, and ones that I can answer," her doctor responds. "I'll start by answering your last question: it's never too late to start exercising. You can gain the health benefits from exercising at any age."

"Well, that's good to hear," Sue says with relief.

Wondering if you are too old to start exercising? The good news is that whether you are forty-nine or ninety-four, you're at a great age to start exercising. There are many studies that show even if you have been sedentary all your life, you're never too old to start making exercise part of your routine. Perhaps you were physically active in your teen years but became too busy for sports and exercise as you became older. Given the benefits of staying physically active, it is important to try to find ways to engage in exercise even when your life is busy. It is never too late to start an exercise routine and reap the benefits.

CHECK WITH YOUR DOCTOR PRIOR TO STARTING A NEW EXERCISE PROGRAM AND IF YOU ARE HAVING ANY NEW OR CONCERNING SYMPTOMS WHEN EXERCISING

"I'm glad you wanted to check in with me prior to starting to exercise. We can plan an exercise program together that can help your body and mind while minimizing the risks of exercising."

"There are risks of exercising?" Sue asks, surprised.

"Yes. Most people never run into any trouble, but if you haven't exercised regularly before (or not for a long time), we should make sure that your heart, lungs, muscles, joints, and other parts of your body are prepared for the exercise, and also that you know the warning signs when the exercise might actually be harming your body."

Sue and her doctor go over some of the warning signs.

"Wow, I never knew I would need to worry about all those things!"

"There isn't really anything to 'worry' about. Most of the things I'm mentioning are just common sense—don't do something if it causes you pain, discomfort, or other problems."

"OK, that makes sense."

"Good. Let's spend a few minutes reviewing why exercise is good for your brain and the rest of your body, and then we'll chat about the specifics of which exercises are best for you and how much you should be doing. How does that sound?"

"It sounds great," Sue says, smiling.

After going through some of the reasons that exercise is good for the body and brain, Sue and her doctor review different types of exercise and decide that brisk walking thirty minutes each day plus a yoga class twice a week is best for her.

It is important for you to check with your doctor before starting a brand-new exercise program. Checking with your doctor is especially critical if you have a family history of heart disease, are a current or former smoker, are overweight, or have any of the following conditions: high cholesterol, high blood pressure, diabetes or prediabetes (high blood sugars), asthma or other lung disease, arthritis, or kidney disease. Lastly, if you experience any of the following warning signs when you are exercising, you should seek immediate medical attention by calling your doctor or dialing 911 (in most regions of the United States): pain or discomfort in your chest, neck, jaw, arms, or legs; dizziness or fainting; shortness of breath; ankle swelling; rapid heartbeat; leg pain; or other symptoms you are concerned about.

AN IDEAL EXERCISE PROGRAM INCLUDES AT LEAST THIRTY MINUTES DAILY OF AEROBIC EXERCISE PLUS ADDITIONAL EXERCISE FOR STRENGTH, BALANCE, AND FLEXIBILITY EACH WEEK

The Centers for Disease Control, American Congress of Sports Medicine, and the National Institutes of Health all agree that the minimum recommended amount of exercise is thirty minutes of moderate aerobic activity on most—and optimally all— days each week. Aerobic exercise is any activity that gets you breathing harder and gets your heart beating faster. An example of moderate aerobic activity is taking a brisk walk. Too busy for a thirty-minute walk? Research also suggests that shorter bursts of exercise, just ten minutes at a time, can also improve overall health if these bursts accumulate to at least thirty minutes each day. Although the majority of research has focused on the benefits of aerobic exercise, there is also evidence that resistance training contributes to a modest improvement in many vascular risk factors. We recommend two sessions of strength training a week, which can improve balance and muscle function and can even reduce age-related brain shrinkage and holes in the brain's white matter (the wiring between different brain regions).

For the vast majority of older adults, there is some form of safe physical activity that can be identified even in the presence of seemingly significant obstacles. For example, individuals with leg amputations can engage—and excel—in highly demanding sports. Even those individuals unable to stand can perform a *sitting* exercise program that provides a very vigorous workout (trust us, we've taken it!). There is an exercise program out there for just about everyone. In addition to walking, you can use a bicycle or one of the machines available at fitness clubs and YMCAs, such as a treadmill, stationary bike, elliptical machine, and StairMaster. Walking in a shallow pool and swimming are also great ways to get aerobic exercise and are some of the best forms of exercise if you are having any pain in your joints, such as arthritis. If you are participating in sports such as tennis, golf, hockey, or skiing, keep those activities going! Lastly, note that there has been no identified point of diminishing returns when it comes to exercise and brain health—the more the better. As long as your heart, joints, muscles, and other parts of your body are OK with even more exercise than thirty minutes a day, consider doing more.

EXERCISE REDUCES THE RISK OF STROKES

As we discussed in Chapters 6 and 9, cardiovascular disease and medical conditions such as diabetes, high blood pressure, high cholesterol, heart disease, and obesity can contribute to memory loss due to strokes. A sedentary lifestyle is one of the major risk factors for the development of strokes. Exercise can help minimize and even eliminate many of the conditions that are considered risk factors for strokes. Exercise helps promote weight loss, which can reduce the risk of stroke for those who are overweight and obese. In fact, compared to adults who maintain a healthy weight, overweight adults are 22 percent more likely to suffer a stroke and obese adults are 64 percent more likely. Additional benefits of exercise for cardiovascular health include lowering blood pressure and total cholesterol by lowering "bad" cholesterol (LDL) and raising "good" cholesterol (HDL). Adults who exercise lower their risk of diabetes and even those with diabetes show better control over blood sugars.

FALLS ARE MORE COMMON WITH AGE

Sue leaves the doctor's office building, holding onto the railing as she carefully goes down the stairs. As she walks through the parking lot, her foot catches on some uneven pavement. She stumbles forward and almost falls.
I've got to be more careful when I walk, Sue says to herself.

The risk of falling increases as we age. In fact, one out of every three adults over age sixty-five falls each year. Walking downstairs can be hazardous—particularly if your hands are full so that you cannot hold onto the railing or see where your feet are stepping. Uneven pavement or ground can often cause a fall when one isn't expecting it. Of those adults who experience a fall, 20 to 30 percent suffer moderate to severe consequences, such as hip fracture or head injury. Head injuries due to falls can result in permanent cognitive impairment or even death.

YOGA AND TAI CHI CAN REDUCE FALLS

Sue knows that she never had very good balance and getting older has not improved it. *Well*, she sighs to herself, *yoga is supposed to improve balance . . . I might as well give it a try.*
Sue joins an introductory yoga class, borrowing a mat from the studio.
"We'll start in child's pose," the teacher instructs. "Spread your knees apart and bring your toes to touch, resting your buttocks on your heels. Bow forward, arms extended long, palms down, allow your forehead to come to your mat. Soften and relax your lower back. Allow all tension in your shoulders, arms, and neck to drain away. Keep your gaze inward with your eyes closed. Focus on your breath. Let your thoughts drift away."

The class continues. Additional poses are introduced: downward dog, forward fold, halfway lift, table top, warrior two, crescent lunge, and many others. The teacher comes by and helps her with a pose, evening her hips, extending her arms. She has difficulty with many poses and she finds her body is quite stiff. . . .

Six weeks have gone by, and she has continued in the class twice a week. She's now much better at the poses and, to her surprise, she finds that she is more flexible and has better balance. Because she isn't struggling with the poses, she's been able to concentrate on her breathing, which has helped her to be more relaxed and less anxious. She's also made some new friends.

Walking out of class, she catches her sandal on a concrete lip that was higher than the others. She is afraid that she will fall. To her surprise, she doesn't even stumble. Her body—knowing what to do without instructions—simply supports herself on her other leg while she regains her balance. She smiles and walks to her car with a more confident stride.

About half of all falls can be prevented with an exercise program that works to increase muscle strength, bone stability, and balance, such as Tai Chi and yoga. For the best results, practice such programs at least two hours weekly, which averages just over fifteen minutes each day.

EXERCISE IMPROVES SLEEP

In addition to participating in yoga twice weekly, Sue is gradually increasing her daily walking. She began with fifteen minutes a day and, increasing by five minutes every other week, she is now up to thirty minutes daily except on her yoga days.

"I don't know about all this exercise," she complains to John. "After I finish a thirty-minute brisk walk, I feel so fatigued that I need to rest for another thirty minutes!"

"There's nothing wrong with that," John says. "That's how you know you got a good workout. And besides, you're ramping up your exercise and your body is still getting used to the level of activity."

Later that night Sue crawls into bed beside John. "Well, there is one good thing about all this exercise," she says aloud. "I now can fall asleep the instant my head hits the pillow. It is hard to even imagine that I used to need sleeping pills . . . exercise is definitely better than all of them!"

As we discussed in Step 5, Chapter 13, sleep is critically important for memory. If you are tired you won't be able to pay attention to what is going on around you, and if you cannot pay attention well, you won't be able to remember well either. We also know that the process of memories going from short-term, temporary storage to a more permanent, long-term storage requires sleep. We sleep best when we go through different sleep stages, including dream sleep and deep sleep. As we age, those stages are not as strong or as long as they used to be. In addition, conditions like insomnia and sleep apnea affect more older adults than younger adults. Exercise is one way to help improve sleep. For older adults complaining of a sleep disturbance, beginning an exercise program results in improvements in the quality of sleep, the amount of time it takes to fall asleep, and the number of times one wakes during the night. Beneficial effects begin after several months of exercising consistently. In addition, exercise reduces the need to rely on medication to assist with sleep. Thus, exercise can be used to improve sleep and may be an alternative or complement to medication management of sleep disorders.

EXERCISE IMPROVES MOOD

I'm really looking forward to my walk today, Sue thinks to herself. It's been about three months since Sue started exercising and she has finally reached her target exercise regimen: walking briskly thirty minutes each day plus an hour of yoga twice weekly.

Sue has discovered that she often runs into friends and neighbors on her walks, and she enjoys stopping and catching up with them when she sees them. But she always notes the time that she paused and resumed her walking on her watch so that she makes sure she gets her full thirty minutes of exercise in.

Sue feels energetic and full of life. *Wow,* she thinks, *I never really thought I would be doing this much exercise—and enjoying it.*

As we learned in Step 4, Chapter 12, memory can be negatively impacted by a number of emotional factors, including anxiety and depression. Exercise has been shown to decrease depression and anxiety and also brighten mood—even in people who don't have anxiety and depression. (Everyone could benefit from being a little happier, right?) Often this mood-boosting effect occurs within minutes of engaging in exercise, providing some immediate gratification. Exercise increases levels of serotonin and norepinephrine—important brain chemicals—and teaches our bodies how to deal more effectively with physical and psychological stress. Exercise can help people who are isolated socialize more. Exercise can also give you a sense of accomplishment. Exercise may improve your appearance and make you feel better about your physical attractiveness. All of these things can help reduce depression and anxiety. In fact, exercise has been found to be as effective as medication in treating depression and anxiety.

EXERCISE RELEASES GROWTH FACTORS THAT PRODUCE NEW BRAIN CELLS

Sue is out enjoying her daily walk, this time with a friend who has been joining her each Tuesday. They discuss politics, sports, national news, local events in their community, books, and their families. They walk along in silence for a few minutes, enjoying the beauty of the leaves starting to turn color at the beginning of autumn.

I haven't noticed any problems with my memory recently, Sue thinks to herself as she walks. *I can recall recent news events, names of family and friends, books I've read, and movies I've seen. Maybe this exercise is helping my brain.*

We discussed in Steps 1 and 2 that the hippocampus is the memory center of the brain that forms and stores new memories. In addition to improving thinking and memory by contributing to the physical health of the body and the emotional health of the mind, exercise can also directly affect brain structure. There are growth factors in the brain that are critical for the survival of brain cells. Without enough of these growth factors, brain cells die, whereas when their levels increase, our brain can produce new cells. Exercise increases the level of these factors, promoting the growth of new brain cells and the health of existing cells, particularly in the hippocampus. The hippocampus tends to be larger in fit older adults compared to those with lower fitness levels. In addition, aerobic exercise training can increase the size of the hippocampus in older adults, with one study finding as much as a 2 percent increase in the size of the hippocampus— equal to reversing aging in the brain by one to two years! Even those with a family history of Alzheimer's disease dementia can gain important benefits. One particularly exciting study examined the size of the hippocampus in cognitively healthy older adults with the gene APOE-e4 that increases the risk of

Alzheimer's disease before and after starting an exercise program. After a year and half, they found that the hippocampus had shrunk about 3 percent in those older adults who did not exercise, whereas those who engaged in a consistent exercise routine experienced almost no shrinkage of the hippocampus.

EXERCISE IMPROVES THINKING AND MEMORY IN HEALTHY INDIVIDUALS

The majority of studies that have examined the relationship between exercise and cognitive functioning have found that engaging in exercise on a regular basis is associated with the maintenance of cognitive health and prevention of cognitive decline as one ages. Other studies found that the more often and more strenuously you exercise, the greater are your gains in thinking and memory. The benefits of exercise on thinking and memory have been found for both those who have been exercising lifelong and those who are just starting to exercise. These findings mean that if you are already an exerciser and have been for much of your life—good for you!—you are already getting the benefits that exercise provides for brain health. It also means that if you aren't currently an exerciser or you don't exercise as much as you'd like to—no problem—you can start today and reap the benefits that exercise offers for the brain. Lastly, the effects of exercise are cumulative over years, so that each year you exercise regularly increases its benefit.

EXERCISE IMPROVES THINKING, MEMORY, AND QUALITY OF LIFE IN INDIVIDUALS WITH MILD COGNITIVE IMPAIRMENT AND DEMENTIA DUE TO ALZHEIMER'S DISEASE

For those diagnosed with mild cognitive impairment (see Step 3, Chapter 7), exercise can improve thinking and memory in as little as six months. One study in people with mild cognitive impairment found that improvements in thinking and memory due to exercise were related to greater efficiency when performing cognitive tasks. For those older adults diagnosed with dementia due to Alzheimer's disease (see Step 3, Chapters 7 and 8), exercising regularly can lead to improved thinking, memory, and quality of life for individuals and their care partners. Mood, agitation, and irritability are all improved with exercise in those with dementia. Importantly, exercise also helps preserve functioning in daily life in those with Alzheimer's disease dementia.

MAKE AN EXERCISE PLAN

Despite the numerous beneficial effects that exercise has on physical, emotional, and brain health, most adults do not get an adequate amount of exercise. In fact, less than one-third of adults in America get the minimum recommended amount of physical activity. It is estimated that between one-third and one-half of people over the age of seventy-five engage in no leisure time physical activity at all. Some of the most common barriers to exercise reported by older adults include factors related to health concerns (such as physical disability, fear of injury) and environmental barriers (such as weather, presence/ quality of sidewalks). Make an exercise plan and begin slowly with small exercise goals you feel confident you can accomplish and build from there. Make goals specific. For example, instead of saying, "I'm going to exercise more this week," you should specify what that means, as in, "I'm going to walk three days this week for thirty minutes each day." Have alternative plans for inclement weather such as walking in the mall or on a treadmill. Find exercises you enjoy and make them part of your daily routine so your commitment to exercise can be lifelong.

SUMMARY

Exercise can strengthen your memory and your thinking. Exercise improves your physical health by increasing cardiovascular fitness, promoting weight loss, improving sleep, and reducing the risk of strokes and falls. Exercise also improves your mood by releasing neurotransmitter brain chemicals that can make you feel good. In addition, exercise releases growth factors in your brain that can enhance your thinking and memory whether your memory is normal or not—and the release of these growth factors can even increase the size of your brain!

We encourage you to create an exercise program that is right for you. Form a realistic plan and make it part of your daily routine. Lastly, it is important to go over your exercise plan with your doctor to make sure that it is a good plan for your overall health. Remember, it's never too late to start exercising!

Let's now consider some examples to illustrate what we learned in this chapter.

- You know that exercise is good for you, but you are sure you get enough exercise just from doing your daily chores. Every day you do laundry, vacuum, and wash the dishes. You also pick the grandkids up from school. With all of that running around, surely you don't need to exercise any more, right?
  - Well, not exactly. Doing household chores is better than doing nothing at all, but most people overestimate how much aerobic exercise they get from household chores alone. Most household chores do not give you the kind of workout you need to benefit the brain. You should aim for moderate intensity when exercising. That is a perceived exertion of 5 or 6 on a scale of 1 to 10, where 0 is sitting and 10 is working as hard as you can.
- Your friend tells you all about the benefits of exercise over lunch, but you aren't sure what type of exercise you should be doing or how much.
  - The minimum recommended activity is thirty minutes of moderate exercise five days each week. The exercise should be

aerobic, meaning that it gets you breathing hard and your blood pumping. It is best to pick something that you enjoy so you will keep doing it. Popular activities include walking, running, biking, swimming, and dancing. Some people need to take medical issues or disability into consideration when selecting an activity.

- You know all about the ways in which exercise benefits the brain, and you would really love to exercise, but you have a heart condition. What should you do?
  o All older adults should consult their physician before beginning an exercise program, especially when one has medical conditions such as heart disease, diabetes, high blood pressure, arthritis, or asthma. For the majority of adults, there is some form of safe exercise.
- You want to exercise and you've even tried to start an exercise routine a couple of times before. Unfortunately, you are just too busy, and every time you begin a new routine, you eventually give up. You just can't find the time.
  o If your schedule is too busy to find a large chunk of time to exercise, try breaking it up into smaller units, such as three ten-minute periods. For example, you can park your car further away from the office in the morning and take a brisk ten-minute walk to and from work. You can take a walk during lunch or after dinner. It's easier than you think to fit in brief exercise programs throughout your day.

Step 6

STRENGTHEN
YOUR MEMORY

In Step 5 we learned about the changes you can make in your sleep, diet, and level of physical activity to help improve your memory and reduce the risk of Alzheimer's disease and its effects. In Step 6 we will discuss how to strengthen your memory in daily life. We first discuss the use of mental exercises: pencil-and-paper games and drills as well as computerized memory training. Do such activities make you smarter and improve your thinking and memory? Are there other activities that do? Next, we discuss the strategies that you can use to improve your memory performance. Lastly, we discuss the aids that are available to improve your memory function in everyday life.

16

What Can I Do to Strengthen My Memory?

We are often asked if there are mental exercises that people can do to help them remain sharp and stave off memory loss. What about online or computer brain-training games that are currently being sold with promises to improve memory and the health of the brain? Is it true that doing crossword puzzles, Sudoku, and similar activities will keep the brain young and prevent memory loss? Are there other mental activities you should be doing to keep your brain healthy? We explore these questions in this chapter.

BRAIN-TRAINING GAMES: NOT ENOUGH EVIDENCE—YET

Jack and his daughter, Sara, have gotten into a little argument. Sara has purchased a subscription to an online, computerized brain-training program. She would like Jack to spend at least thirty minutes each day working on it.

"Can you just try it, Dad?" Sara asks with exasperation.

"I don't like those things, Sara," Jack exclaims. "I'm no good at computers. It was computers that lost me my job. I know that you are a wiz at this computer stuff, but I'm not. Computers make me feel old and stupid."

"I'm not asking you to become an expert," Sara says. "I'd just like you to try it. The website says it can make you smarter and make your brain younger. Here, let me show you . . ." She clicks through several screens on the computer. "OK," she continues, "I guess it doesn't actually *say* it will make your brain younger, but it implies it right here." She points to some text on the screen.

"Sara, I know you're trying to help me, but I want to go to that pottery class so I can finish my project, and then I'm meeting the guys to play hockey. I don't have time for this computer stuff."

"Can't you miss your hockey game for one week? And your 'hockey' game seems more like a social event anyways—you spend one hour playing and two hours chatting over dinner."

"So, what's wrong with that? We have dinner together after playing, and I'm working on eating better—just like you showed me."

"Can't you just try the computer?"

Jack looks at Sara defiantly, but then sees in her eyes how much she is trying to help him. He softens his gaze. "OK. For you, Sara, I'll give it a try. But I'm still going to go to the pottery class and then to play hockey with the guys."

"Thanks, Dad. That's all I'm asking. Please give it a try."

Making sure he is on the right page of the website, Sara leaves her father to the computer training. Jack looks at the clock. *OK,* he thinks to himself, *I can spend ten minutes on this computer stuff and still have time to go to the pottery class and get ready for hockey.* Jack completes the first set of exercises on the computer. *Well, it wasn't as bad as I thought, although I don't feel any smarter . . .*

The brain-training anti-aging industry is among the fastest growing industries in the marketplace, with current annual revenues estimated at $3.2 billion and forecast to increase to more than $15 billion over the next several years. But do these products really work? That question has been under hot debate for some time. In 2016 the Federal Trade Commission decided that certain products made exaggerated claims, and this agency imposed fines and ordered the removal of unsubstantiated claims from products' advertising materials. It is true that certain brain-training products have shown some promise in research, but the results have been mixed. These products often show that people make gains on the trained task, but the gains do not generalize to other aspects of day-to-day functioning. People also often report feeling better about the health of their brains, but there is little evidence that actual improvements in brain fitness occur. So, when you play brain-training games, you may get better at playing the game and you may feel better about the health of your brain, but unfortunately that feeling doesn't translate into real improvement in brain health. In short, there is not currently strong enough evidence for us to suggest the use of brain-training games.

Similarly, although it can be enjoyable to challenge yourself with crossword puzzles, Sudoku, and other games, these forms of entertainment have not been shown to significantly impact brain aging. Again, doing these types of puzzles may make you better at doing them, but they are not likely to improve the overall health of your brain. (Note, however, that these activities are better for the brain than watching TV.) Our advice: If you want to do brain training and puzzles because you find them enjoyable, go ahead, but if you are doing these things in the hopes of improving your memory, then save your time and money. Having stated that clearly, we would add that there has been an explosion of new products that are being designed and tested—some with the help of doctors and scientists—so there may be beneficial products available in the future.

If these activities don't help to promote the health of the brain, what does? We recommend that you engage in activities that keep you mentally stimulated, socially active, and foster a positive mental attitude toward aging (and life in general). Many of these activities may also promote physical exercise, which—as you learned in Step 5, Chapter 15—is vitally important in keeping the brain healthy.

ENGAGE IN NOVEL, MENTALLY STIMULATING ACTIVITIES

"Make sure you've wet your hands a little, and then start working with the clay," explains the instructor.

Jack is at his local crafts store where he is attending a class on making pottery. Jack pays close attention. An electrician all his life, the closest thing he has done to pottery has been using plaster and spackle to repair walls and ceilings. Now he is trying to make a vase for Sara.

"The walls shouldn't be too thick or too thin," continues the instructor. "Work to create a uniform thickness in your piece."

Jack is struggling to achieve uniform thickness. "Hey," Jack says, turning to a man in his fifties sitting on his left, "how did you get such a nice, smooth thickness?"

"Try this tool, and use a bit more water—your clay is too dry."

"Right," Jack responds. "Thanks, I keep forgetting about the water."

Between the water and the tool Jack's piece is back on track.

"Hey, that's looking like a nice vase!"

"Thanks," Jack responds. "Your bowl looks great, too."

"How are you liking the class?"

"It's both harder and more fun than I thought it would be," answers Jack. "What about you?"

"Agree completely. Now that my kids are out of the house it gives me something to do—other than watch TV—while my wife is at her book club."

Engaging in novel, mentally stimulating activities can reduce your risk of dementia. Which mentally stimulating activities are best? Activities that provide novel experiences, such as learning a new skill, taking up a new hobby, and visiting a new place, lead to the most gains in brain health. Doing something new that stretches you outside of your comfort zone appears to be most beneficial. Less stimulating activities— such as watching television—may actually *increase* your risk of developing dementia. Many mentally stimulating activities also provide social stimulation or physical activity; the benefits are clearly greatest when you engage in all three types of activities—mental, social, and physical. So rather than investing in online or computerized brain games, crossword puzzles, Sudoku, or the like, we recommend that you engage in complex, novel, mentally stimulating activities: attend a community education class, learn a new hobby, or take up a new sport.

PURSUE SOCIAL ACTIVITIES

Jack and his friend Sam have just finished playing hockey with their teammates. In the Introduction we learned that Sam, whose wife has dementia, expressed concern about Jack's memory, starting him down the path to get his memory checked out.

"Not bad tonight for a bunch of old-timers!" Jack exclaims. He is in the locker room of the skating rink changing back into his street clothes.

"Absolutely!" Sam agrees. "That was a great pass you gave me!"

"That was a great goal you scored with my pass!" says Jack.

"It's all about teamwork," Sam replies.

"Too bad we lost six to one."

"Well, you win some, you lose some . . ."

"Or in our case, you lose some, you lose some!"

Sam smiles.

Jack and Sam walk out of the skating rink with their teammates
and go to the local restaurant across the street. They move
to their usual table in the back of the room, saying hello
to and chatting with the other regulars in the restaurant as
they go.

"Ahh," Jack sighs as he eases his sore body into the booth.
"It's always good to relax here after the game," he says to
his six hockey-playing friends as they also crowd into the
round booth.

Everyone nods and several make their own groaning noises as
they sit down.

The server comes over to take their drink order. "You guys
all want your usuals?" she asks. Everyone nods or grunts
a "yes."

"I've got the first round," Jack says to the server, "put them on
my tab."

When the drinks come back, Jack raises his glass for a toast,
"To some of the worst hockey players—and best group of
friends a guy could have!"

Humans are social animals. Our social relationships continue
to be important as we age—so important, in fact, that our social
experiences help our brains age successfully. Unfortunately,
many adults face threats to socialization as they age, such as
retirement, widowhood, and loss of friends and family members, which can result in a shrinking social network. The proportion of older adults living alone increases with advancing
age. Pandemics may also increase social isolation when individuals are advised to limit contact with others to avoid catching potentially dangerous infections. Loneliness, the feeling of
being lonely regardless of living arrangements, may affect more
than 40 percent of older adults and has been associated with
cognitive decline. Low social participation, less frequent social
contact, and loneliness have all been associated with the onset
of dementia.

By contrast, participating in social activities has been shown to have cognitive benefits. One large study following over 1,000 older adults for five years found that those who were the most socially active showed 70 percent less cognitive decline than those with the lowest rates of social activity. Note that the quality of social activity matters. Negative social interactions have been associated with cognitive decline.

To benefit brain health and overall well-being, we recommend that you seek out social opportunities as you age, focusing on the cultivation of positive relationships and the reduction of negative social interactions. Local community centers, clubs, and lodges; churches, synagogues, and mosques; continuing education centers, sports leagues, and yoga classes; and many other organizations present opportunities for increasing socialization. In addition, many of these organizations' activities provide mental stimulation or physical activity that, as discussed above, can also improve brain health.

KEEP A POSITIVE MENTAL ATTITUDE

Jack, Sam, and their buddies on the hockey team are relaxing in the booth at the restaurant after finishing their entrees. Jack had the fish and mixed vegetables.

"You know the thing I like best about playing hockey?" Jack asks.

"You get to skate around on the ice with a bunch of sweaty old farts?" one of his friends answers.

"No," Jack responds, smiling. "What I like best is that I say to myself, 'Jack, if you can still play hockey, you can't be that old.'"

"Yeah," Sam chimes in, "I know what you mean. When I play I forget my age . . . although I remember it the next morning when I wake up so sore I can barely move!"

"I agree," says another friend at the table, "although being sore the next morning is a good thing—proves you played hard—and I've been feeling sore after hockey since I was a kid."

"Speaking of kids," says a third friend, "what makes me feel young is chasing after my grandkids. Makes me feel like a new father again."

"Definitely," Sam agrees, "but the best part about grandkids is that you get to give them back at the end of the day."

Jack smiles. "I feel the same way when I'm with my grand-daughter. It's just like I'm thirty years old again. Sometimes I think it's true what they say: You're as young as you feel."

"Attitude is a little thing that makes a big difference." This quotation by Winston Churchill captures the findings of an emerging body of research that suggests that your attitude toward aging can play an important role in how well you age. When older adults were shown negative words about aging, such as decrepit and senile, they actually performed worse on tests of memory, thinking, and physical function compared to when they were shown positive words about aging, such as wise and experienced. One long-term study found that over a thirty-eight-year period, people who held more positive views about aging showed 30 percent less decline in their memory compared with those who held more negative views. We are not saying that having a positive attitude alone can cure diseases of the brain, but having a positive attitude can improve your emotional well-being and influence the way you behave as you age. If you have more positive views about aging, you are more likely to engage in behaviors that promote the health of the brain, like exercising, eating a nutritious diet, and taking medication as prescribed. Cultivating a positive attitude can be as simple as not buying into old-age stereotypes and resisting the urge to make negative comments about your own aging. Recognize and appreciate that your age and experience have given you wisdom that you can share with others. Seek out and spend more time with successful agers you know. Focus on the positive aspects of your life.

SUMMARY

"Thanks so much, Dad, it's beautiful," Sara says after Jack gives her the now completed vase from pottery class. "It will look perfect here on the kitchen table."

She pauses, looking at bit more serious, and says, "You know, Dad . . ."

"I know what you're going to ask me about," Jack interrupts defensively, "you want to know if I've been doing those brain-training computer games. I've done some—honestly. It's just hard to find the time with the other activities I've been doing: the pottery class, playing hockey and, yes, hanging out with the guys. Maybe it's not as good as the computer stuff, but I like doing those things. It makes me feel young—or at least not quite so old."

Sara starts again. "Yes, what I was going to say is that there was an article in the newspaper the other day that suggested that, in fact, all the things that you are doing—learning a new hobby, exercising vigorously, spending time on social activities, and keeping a positive mental attitude—are actually better than the computerized brain-training exercises. In fact," Sara continues sheepishly, "it turns out that there is actually very little evidence that these computer exercises actually help."

"Does that mean I don't have to do them anymore?" Jack asks hopefully.

"Yes," Sara replies, smiling. "Just keep doing all those other things you're doing—those are the best things for your brain."

There is currently not enough evidence for online and computerized brain-training games to justify the investment of time and money. Engaging in mentally stimulating activities— particularly those that are novel and challenging such as learning a new hobby—may be beneficial for brain health. Lastly, social activities and having a positive mental attitude about aging can improve emotional well-being and provide the motivation needed to make healthy lifestyle changes (such as exercising and eating healthy) that can improve memory, thinking, and brain health.

Let's now consider some examples to illustrate what we learned in this chapter.

- You've heard the advertisements for online and computerized brain-training games. Should you buy them to improve your memory?
  o Research into online and computerized brain-training products generally fails to demonstrate gains in real-world functioning. People who use these types of games usually improve at playing the game and often report feeling better about the health of their brain, but there is not good evidence that memory, the health of the brain, or daily functioning actually improves. We suggest engaging in other types of activities that keep you mentally stimulated, socially engaged, and physically active.
- You have heard the old saying "Use it or lose it" applied to brain health. You know you should be staying mentally active, but you aren't sure what that means.
  o Studies suggest that engaging in novel, complex, mentally stimulating activities is a good way to promote the health of your brain. Learning a new skill, taking up a new hobby, visiting a new place, and learning a new language are all examples of complex, novel activities. Local colleges and universities, senior centers, and continuing education programs are good places to look for activities that may interest you.
- You do crossword puzzles and Sudoku every day. Will these activities help to protect your brain?
  o Doing crossword puzzles and Sudoku will improve your ability to do crossword puzzles and Sudoku. There is no evidence that they will improve the overall health of your brain. If you enjoy these activities, by all means keep doing them! If you are only doing them to protect your brain, then we suggest you consider

other activities that are complex and novel and offer added opportunity for socialization and/or physical exercise.

- Ever since you retired you have been less socially active and often feel lonely. Will this affect the health of your brain?
  - o It can. Loneliness has been associated with cognitive decline, whereas remaining socially active has been associated with cognitive benefits. We recommend that you actively seek out ways to remain engaged socially. Join social groups and make regular plans with family and friends.
- You don't see the point in trying to make changes to improve the health of your brain. You are convinced that no matter what you do, your memory will get worse as you get older, so why bother?
  - o As we learned in Step 1, Chapter 2, there are some changes in thinking and memory that are normal as we age, but memory loss related to Alzheimer's or another disease is not. Negative beliefs about aging may actually influence how well you care for yourself and your brain as you age. Don't buy into ageist stereotypes. Resist the urge to make negative comments about your own aging. Look for examples of successful agers. Remain positive about aging.

17

What Strategies Can I Use to Help My Memory?

There are a number of different strategies or tricks that you can use to improve your memory in everyday life. Memory strategies take effort and motivation to use. Some you may already use, some you may know about but not use, and others may be new to you. At first, using a new strategy may seem awkward and you may not be entirely successful, but the more you practice, the more automatic using the strategy will become and the easier it will be to apply. Many strategies work best when used in combination—you'll see that as we describe the strategies in this chapter. Note that not every strategy works for every person. We recommend you try them all and then pick the ones you like. We encourage you to be creative: develop new ways to apply strategies or invent entirely new strategies that work best for you.

PRACTICE ACTIVE ATTENTION

Sue is enjoying her twice-weekly yoga class and daily walks with friends. She has just finished an adult education course that teaches people of any age strategies to improve their memory in daily life. Sue was surprised (and relieved) to find out that many people have difficulty remembering things, even those who are much younger than her. Now she is working hard to put these strategies into practice while on a trip to London.

After an uneventful flight, she and John are heading to the Underground to go to their hotel. There are many over-head announcements, which they are ignoring. They finally reach the Underground platform. They are waiting for about twenty minutes.

"Do you think something is wrong?" Sue asks John.

"Yes, must be," John replies.

An overhead announcement comes on: "For travelers trying to reach London via the Piccadilly line . . ."

"John!" Sue exclaims, "I think that's the Underground line we need to take. We need to listen to that announcement!"

John nods, and they wait as they listen to a stream of other overhead announcements.

I know what I need to do, Sue says to herself. *I need to focus and practice active attention, just like I learned in class.* Sue can begin to feel her heart beating faster. *Don't get nervous*, she tells herself.

"For travelers trying to reach London via the Piccadilly line . . . ," begins the overhead announcement. "Proceed to the central bus station between terminals . . ."

"Did you catch that?" John asks.

"No," replies Sue, "I missed it, too. Give me a minute; I'll get it next time it comes on."

You can do this, Sue tells herself. She spends a minute focusing on slow, deep breaths, using her yoga techniques to calm herself. She feels her heart slowing back down.

"For travelers trying to reach London via the Piccadilly line," begins the overhead announcement again.

Here we go, Sue, focus! she says to herself with determination. Closing her eyes and blocking out other distractions with her mind, she listens to each word, focusing all of her

attention on the announcement. Sue pictures each step of
the detour in her mind as it is spoken.

"I've got it," Sue says, pleased with herself. "We need to go to
the central bus station, between terminals 2 and 3. There
we take the bus to Hatton Cross where we can get on the
Piccadilly line toward Cockfosters, which goes through central London."

"Wow, Sue . . ." John begins.

"Thanks, but give me a minute," Sue interrupts. "I want to
repeat the directions to myself a few more times."

In Step 1 we learned that the frontal lobes need to pay attention to what is coming in from the senses in order to bring
information in from the outside world and send it to the
hippocampus to be bound into a new memory that can be
retrieved later. We discussed that anyone, of any age, can
have difficulty paying attention, and also that older frontal
lobes may require additional effort to pay attention. Often
our frontal lobes are distracted and do not give full attention
to the information we are receiving. For example, we may
be listening to a news story and also worrying about all the
errands we need to do during the day. We may be parking
our car and also thinking about the stores we want to visit
or the appointment we are about to have. In these examples,
we are likely to "forget" the news story or where we parked
because we were not really paying attention to those things
in the first place.

Our first strategy to improve our memory is to *practice
active attention*. When we use passive attention, we simply
allow information to be presented to us without making a
conscious effort to process or learn that information. When
we use active attention, we try to be fully "in the moment,"
putting effort into taking in the information being presented.
For example, when listening to a news story that you'd like

to remember for later, you can notice how you feel about the story, what its implications are, and what questions it raises. Similarly, when you are parking your car, make it a point to observe your surroundings and make a mental note of any landmarks. Mindfulness training is one way to learn active attention. It emphasizes, among other things, being "in the moment" and "paying attention on purpose." Studies have shown that practicing mindfulness can improve thinking and memory abilities. If you are interested in learning more about mindfulness training, you can look for classes or teachers in your area or purchase print or audio books that focus on the practice of mindfulness.

MINIMIZE DISTRACTIONS IN THE ENVIRONMENT

In addition to distractions in our mind, such as thoughts and feelings, there are also distractions in our environment that can make it difficult to pay attention. When we want to learn and remember something, we need to make our environment conducive to learning. Although it isn't always possible, try to learn new information in an environment that is quiet, has adequate lighting, and is away from windows if they might tempt you to stare outside. Turn off your telephone, television, radio, and email program. You might place a "Do Not Disturb" sign on your door to discourage others from interrupting you while you are working to learn new material. Getting rid of clutter in your environment eliminates possible distractions and makes it easier to attend to new information you want to learn. Lastly, when you are having an important conversation with a friend or loved one, make sure you aren't trying to multitask and make eye contact. Don't have one eye on the football game when your wife is asking you to listen to her.

TAKE BREAKS

Paying full attention can be hard work. Your frontal lobes can only pay attention for so long before they become fatigued and your attention starts to wane. When you are trying to learn new information, we recommend that you give yourself a break every hour for about ten minutes. If an hour is too long and you notice your attention waning after a shorter period of time, take a short break then. Everyone is different—find out what break schedule works best for you.

REPEAT INFORMATION SPACED OUT OVER TIME

Repetition is an effective way to improve your memory for any material you're trying to learn. Whether it is rereading a news story you want to remember or repeating information you've been told to ensure understanding, repetition is a simple and powerful tool. Repetition works best when it is spaced out over time, rather than all at once. For example, if you want to remember a story you heard on the news so you can tell your husband about it later, instead of repeating it to yourself several times immediately after hearing it, repeat it once or twice after hearing it, then again about thirty minutes later, and again an hour or two after that. If you're trying to remember material for years, spacing it out over days, weeks, and months works best. It is also helpful to speak the information you want to remember aloud. Saying it out loud increases your focus on the information and deepens your engagement with the material.

MAKE CONNECTIONS

After arriving at their hotel via the Underground, Sue and John are out enjoying London. Following a visit to the British

Museum in the morning, they are standing on its broad front steps, discussing where they should go for lunch.

"Excuse me," says a woman about their age with a familiar, American accent. "I didn't mean to eavesdrop, but I heard you were looking for a good place for lunch. You've just got to try The Square Goose. We had a lunch there yesterday."

"Yes," says the man who is with the woman, "it's like British *tapas* . . . you get a lot of small plates so you can try a little of everything."

"Thanks so much," Sue says, "that sounds like a great option."

Sue is thinking to herself, *OK, I need to remember The Square Goose . . . The Square Goose . . . how will I remember it? I know! I will think of the geese that like to sit in our town square back home . . . that's how I'll remember it!*

Our brains are wired to form connections between information. We can capitalize on this natural tendency when we want to learn something new by intentionally linking the new information with something that we already know. Sometimes it can help to pair this technique with the next one, creating visual images.

CREATE VISUAL IMAGES

Sue and John continue to chat with the American couple. "It's nice to hear a familiar accent," says John, "Where are you from?"

"We're from Utah," the woman responds.

Everyone introduces themselves and shakes hands. Sue and John learn that the couple has been in London for a week and has other good restaurant suggestions to share.

"If you like Indian," the woman says, "try the Golden Sitar on Adam Street."

Sue, continuing to use the techniques she learned in class, creates a comical image in her mind of a gold sitar sitting on top of her nephew Adam's head. A small smile creeps into her face as she thinks about it.

"And if you're interested in French food," the man says, "try the Chateau Rouge, on Bow Street."

Sue makes a visual image of a small castle, painted completely red, and tied up with a big red bow, as if it were a present.

"Oh, and that reminds me of a great bakery nearby," says the woman, "the Red Rose Bakery on King Street."

Sue pictures a king with a crown, and in the center of his crown a loaf of bread with a red rose on top.

When it comes to memory, a picture really is worth a thousand words. Many parking garages take advantage of the power of pictures by labeling parking floors with visual images along with numbers. What if there is no picture provided? Make one! Let's say you parked in lot C, row 4. Before you leave your car, you might take a moment to visualize four cats on its hood, helping you to link the letter C and the number 4 with your parking space. Visual imagery is a powerful technique that can be used to improve your memory in everyday life.

PUT IT IN A LOCATION

After lunch, Sue and John travel to the next destination on their route, Buckingham Palace. Along the way they find a cute tourist shop, and Sue looks for gifts for their grandchildren there. Sue has used another method that she learned in class to memorize what each child wants for their souvenir. Picturing her house back home, she had imagined each child in a different part of the house playing with his or her gift. To retrieve the list of gifts, she mentally "walks through" her house and sees what each child is playing with in her mind. She also has the list written down in her purse, but she wants to see how well she can remember it.

OK Sue, she says to herself, here we go. I'm going to walk through the front door. In the foyer I can see little William playing with his new red double-decker bus, so that's the first gift: a red double-decker bus for William. I am now walking into the living room, and I can see Madeline playing with her book of paper dolls and clothes of the royal family at the coffee table. Robbie is standing on the armchair with his right hand up high, flying his World War I airplane around. James Junior is in the family room trying to get the little ball attached to a string into the cup. Lilly is sitting in the dining room with her colonial-style white bonnet on. Mary is in the kitchen helping her mother with her new apron on. Henry is playing in the bathtub with his inflatable ball. Finally, George is in the bedroom putting on his new Dr. Who T-shirt. OK, Sue says as she counts on her fingers— I've got them all!

The Greeks developed the method of location to remember large amounts of information more than 2,000 years ago. You can use this method, too. Start with a place that you are very familiar with, such as your home. In your mind, walk around your home and fill each room (and even each part of each room, such as the sofa, chair, and table) with something that you want to remember. When you want to retrieve the items, you simply walk through your home in your mind and see what you put in each room. Sometimes it helps if you put things where they would normally go—like chocolate pudding in the kitchen. But it can be even more effective if you put things where they don't go—like chocolate pudding handprints all over the white living room sofa; that is harder to forget! You can also use this method to remember things in order if you wish—just walk in your mind from one end of your home to the other, going through each room and each part of the room in the order you would if you were to really walk through it.

USE THE FIRST-LETTER METHOD

After seeing the changing of the guards at Buckingham Palace in the afternoon, Sue and John are making their way back to their hotel room to rest and relax before dinner.

"Sue," John begins, "help me remember that I'd like to pick up some gum and another umbrella after we get off the Underground."

"Sure," Sue responds, "and if we're stopping, I want to get some more toothpaste, Oil of Olay, Kleenex, and mints."

Sue thinks to herself, *Now, how will I remember all of these things . . . maybe if I make an acronym . . . let's see: T(oothpaste), O(il of) O(lay), K(leenex), M(ints), U(mbrella), and G(um) . . . TOOKMUG . . . perfect! TOOK MUG, that's how I'll remember those items!*

The first-letter method involves creating an easily remembered acronym or abbreviation to help you learn and recall information. It is a helpful method because it organizes lengthy information and provides you with a clue when you try to remember it.

Let's do an exercise. Take a minute and see if you can name all the Great Lakes. Good. Now see if you can name all the colors of the rainbow.

Ready for the answers? The five great lakes are Huron, Ontario, Michigan, Erie, and Superior. The colors of the rainbow are Red, Orange, Yellow, Green, Blue, Indigo, Violet. How did you do? Did you use any tricks to try to remember the information?

Many people rely on the first-letter method to recall the Great Lakes and the colors of the rainbow. HOMES is the acronym used to remember the Great Lakes, and ROYGBIV (or Roy G. Biv) is the acronym used to remember the colors of the rainbow in order. You can look for more ways to use acronyms in your everyday life.

USE CHUNKING

After purchasing the gifts for their grandchildren and the items they need for the hotel, Sue and John are out of the British pounds they brought with them. They stop at a bank ATM. Sue inserts her card and enters her four-digit PIN code, but the process stops there with a message telling her to call her bank. Calling her bank she is told that to use her card overseas she needs to enter a different, ten-digit PIN that will be given to her by the computer, twice, when the bank employee hangs up.

Sue is momentarily panicking. *How am I ever going to remember a ten-digit number?* "John," she says aloud, "pull out some paper and a pen. I'm going to give you a ten-digit number to write down in a minute."

"Ten digits," John repeats back, "that's as long as a phone number—with area code!"

That's it! Sue says to herself. *Ten digits is like a phone number. I can chunk the ten digits into three, three, and four, just like an area code, city prefix, and number.*

The computer comes on, "Your overseas PIN code is: 5-4-2-7-6-5-3-1-8-0."

542-765-something, Sue says to herself.

The computer continues, "Again, that number is: 5-4-2-7-6-5-3-1-8-0."

542-765-31-80, Sue says to herself, and then aloud: "542-765-31-80, 542-765-31-80."

"I've got it!" John responds triumphantly.

Chunking is a helpful memory tool because it allows you to make a large amount of information smaller and more manageable. Here's an example. Imagine trying to remember these letters:

CIAFBINBACNNABCNFL

Now imagine trying to remember these letters:

CIA-FBI-NBA-CNN-ABC-NFL

Chunking can be useful when you are trying to remember new phone numbers, your license plate, or a computer or bank passcode.

CLUSTER INFORMATION BY TOPIC

Clustering is somewhat similar to chunking, except that the material to be remembered is reorganized into groups. For example, imagine you are given the following list of words to remember:

Original List (random order)
- apple
- bear
- banana
- pen
- orange
- lion
- pencil
- marker
- tiger

Now try clustering them into categories:

Clustered List (animals, fruits, writing instruments)
- lion
- tiger
- bear
- apple
- orange
- banana
- pencil
- pen
- marker

Clustering can be used to remember items you need at the supermarket, items you need to bring with you when you leave the house, or errands you need to run during the day. Cluster beauty errands like going to the hairdresser and getting a manicure, food errands like grocery shopping and picking up dessert at the bakery, and car errands like getting gas and a car wash.

INVENT RHYMES

The next day, Sue and John stroll along the Thames. They pass a man wearing a large body placard advertising The Paris Patisserie and saying in a sing-song voice, "London's best bake-er-ey is The Paris Patiss-er-ie! London's best bake-er-ey is The Paris Patiss-er-ie!"

Later in the afternoon they are making their way along the Thames toward the Globe Theatre and are looking for a snack.

"What do you feel like?" John asks Sue.

"I confess," Sue begins, "that ever since we passed that man advertising The Paris Patisserie I cannot get that jingle out of my head: 'London's best bake-er-ey is The Paris Patiss-er-ie . . .' I'd like to give it a try!"

"Sure, why not . . ." John agrees. "I'll see if I can find one around here."

Try to fill in the blanks for these ad campaigns:

"Don't get mad, get _____."

"Fill it to the rim with _____."

And maybe our favorite, *"Nothing sucks like an _____."*

[Answers: *Glad* (garbage bags), *Brim* (coffee), and *Electrolux* (vacuum)]

Advertisers use rhymes because they work: they are likable and easy to remember. School teachers also use rhymes to help children remember grammatical rules ("i before e except after c") and historical facts ("fourteen hundred ninety-two Columbus sailed the ocean blue"). You can use rhyming in your everyday routines to remember almost any information. For example, "so that I would not be late, I parked my car on level eight," or "before I drive my car ahead, I need to remember to pick up bread."

GET EMOTIONAL

After a delicious treat at The Paris Patisserie, Sue and John reach the Globe Theatre on the Thames. They have seen a number of Shakespeare's plays, but this will be the first time they see *Romeo and Juliet.*

The play begins. Caught up in the passion of the actors, Sue feels she is twenty years old again. When Juliet speaks to Romeo from the balcony, she takes John's hand in hers.

"Good night, good night!" Juliet says to Romeo. "Parting is such sweet sorrow / That I shall say good night till it be morrow."

After the play, Sue and John walk along the Thames, her arm through his, as they make their way back to their hotel.

"What a passionate play!" Sue says. "No wonder it is still being shown 400 years later."

"What was your favorite part?" John asks.

"The balcony scene. I think I'll remember her words forever: 'Parting is such sweet sorrow / That I shall say good night till it be morrow.'"

Do you remember your first kiss? What your date wore to prom? The name of your first pet? Chances are that you can remember some very specific information from a long time ago if that memory was formed during an emotional time in your life. For example, you may be able to remember the weather on the day of your high school graduation but not on a more recent but nonsignificant day. We generally remember information that is emotionally charged better than we remember boring or neutral, nonemotional information for several reasons. We are more likely to pay attention to information that is emotional. We are also more likely to repeat information that is emotional: thinking about the emotional event, playing it over in our minds, and recounting it to others. Additionally, an emotional event activates part of our brain called the amygdala, which tells the hippocampus that this event is important to remember.

So how can you capitalize on emotional memory? When listening to or reading new information, try to engage yourself in the material emotionally. Ask yourself, "How would I feel if I were in that situation?" Attend to the emotional tone of the speaker and your own emotional reactions to the information being presented. Give the information personal, emotional meaning. Have you ever experienced something similar? In this way you are increasing the emotional nature of the information, which will improve your memory for it later.

TEST YOURSELF

Did you ever use flashcards when you needed to study for a test? Then you're already familiar with the benefit of testing yourself when you are learning new information. It has been found that periodically testing yourself on whatever material you are trying to learn is one of the most effective ways to learn new information. When two popular student methods for studying were compared, highlighting and rereading versus making flashcards and self-testing, the self-testing proved to be much more effective. And it turns out that it doesn't matter who makes or administers the test; as long as you're being tested, it will help your memory for the material.

Testing is fairly easy to do. Depending upon what you're trying to learn, you can make flashcards, create a different type of test yourself, or purchase a premade test. You can then test yourself or have someone else quiz you.

WRITE IT DOWN

Another benefit of making flashcards is that by doing so you are writing down the information. People remember information better when they write it down, and, in particular, when they write down the summary or key points of the information, rather than copying it down verbatim. Writing the essence or gist of information requires us to process it deeply, and that deep processing makes us more likely to remember it—even if we never go back and look at our notes.

IT CAN BE DIFFICULT TO REMEMBER NAMES

Sue and John run into the American tourists from Utah whom they had met a week ago, at the Chateau Rouge, one of the restaurants the couple recommended.

"Hi, Sue! Great to see you and John! Have you been enjoying London? I see you took our advice on the restaurants," says the woman.

"Yes and yes—we've been having a great time in London and we really appreciate all of your great restaurant recommendations," Sue says as she is trying hard to recall the name of the woman and her husband.

"You won't be disappointed with this one!" says the man.

Sue is embarrassed that she cannot remember their names, but she plucks up her courage and says, "I'm so sorry that I cannot recall your names—can you remind me?"

Maybe you can relate to this scenario: you're at a party and you spot someone walking toward you. You know you have met him before. Maybe you've met him more than once. Maybe you even remember details about him, such as what he does for work or where he lives. But you can't remember his name. And he is getting closer.

Remembering names deserves its own special section, since it is the most common complaint that older adults have when asked about their memory. There are many things that can interfere with your ability to remember names. Often you may know someone's name but you just can't access it when you need it. In this situation you have learned the name well, but you are having difficulty retrieving it. There can even be a physical sensation of having that name right on the tip of your tongue, and, fittingly, this type of difficulty has been called "tip-of-the-tongue phenomenon" as we discussed in Step 1, Chapter 1. It is also possible that you didn't learn the name well in the first place. Frequently, when we are introduced to people, instead of paying full attention to their names, we are trying to think of what friendly conversation we will make. Or perhaps the problem is that we get introduced to them in the middle of a crowded party with lots of distractions.

WHEN IT IS ON THE TIP OF YOUR TONGUE, RELAX

When you are having trouble retrieving a name you know—when it is on the tip of your tongue—the following strategies might help. First, it is important to try to relax. When you are having this difficulty, you may begin to feel anxious and embarrassed, and these emotions will only make it more difficult to remember the name you are looking for. A few slow deep breaths can often help. Most of these tip-of-the-tongue experiences resolve within a minute or so. Next, try to think of information that you know about the person. What does she do for work? When did you see her last? Where does she live? How do you know her? By thinking of information about him or her that you do know, you are gathering clues to remind you of the name you are looking for. Another technique is to run through the letters of the alphabet looking for the name. There are also things to avoid. Don't repeat a name that sounds like the one you are looking for but isn't it. You may hope that this repetition will trigger the real name, but it usually has the opposite effect—blocking the real name.

LEARN THE NAME WELL IN THE FIRST PLACE

The couple from Utah say their names again for Sue and John. Sue repeats their names out loud and apologizes again for not remembering them.

"Don't worry," says the woman, "we have the same difficulty, too!"

OK, Sue thinks to herself, *now I need to work to connect these names to things I already know so that I won't forget them.*

On the way back to the hotel Sue repeats their names and the connections she has made to remember them a few more times. *I don't know if I'm ever going to see them again,* Sue thinks, *but if I do, I'm going to remember their names!*

The next morning Sue and John head to the airport. To their surprise, standing in the line in front of them are their friends from Utah! It turns out that they are on the same flight back to the United States. This time, without difficulty, Sue is able to greet them both by name.

It is easier to remember names if we make sure we learn them well in the first place. Many of the strategies discussed in this chapter can be applied to learning new names. When you meet someone new, make sure that you heard the name correctly and are paying full attention. Engage your active attention skills. Repeat the name out loud and comment on it, connecting it to something you know: "Oh, your name is Frank? That's also my brother's name!" Use the name when you introduce your-self ("Hi, Frank, my name is John") rather than just stating your own name in return. Engage in visual imagery: imagine the new person in a way that helps recall the name (imagine Frank eating frankfurters). Repeat the name a couple of times throughout the conversation and again when you end the conversation ("Bye, Frank, it was nice meeting you").

Some people may feel uncomfortable repeating someone's name during a conversation—thinking that it sounds like something a salesperson might do. Well, the reason that salespeople do that is because it is helpful for making sales. Repeating the name of someone you meet will help you remember the name—and it also increases the chances that they will like you! So, if you are feeling self-conscious about trying this technique, remind yourself that it's not only good for your memory, it can also help you to make new friends.

REVIEW NAMES PRIOR TO ATTENDING A SOCIAL EVENT

It never hurts to be prepared. Refresh your memory in advance if you know you will be attending an event where friends, acquaintances, or colleagues that you haven't seen for some time will be. You might ask your spouse, a friend, or colleague who they expect to be at the event. You can also use social media sites like Facebook to review the names of people you might expect to see.

IT'S OK TO FORGET A NAME

Sometimes no matter what strategies you use you will forget a name. When this happens, it's okay to be honest. You might say something like, "It's so nice to see you. I remember our last conversation about your daughter very well, but I have to admit that I can't remember your name. Would you remind me?" It is possible—or even likely—that the person you are talking to has forgotten your name, too! Asking for her name might relieve some of her anxiety and provide her with permission to ask you for yours. As we mentioned in the last chapter, keep a positive attitude about aging! If you can't remember someone's name, don't be too hard on yourself. It's common—you're not alone.

SUMMARY

On the flight home Sue enjoys talking with their new friends. Between her daily exercise, increased socializing, and her success in using so many of the memory strategies that she learned in the course, she is feeling less depressed and more confident about her memory.

In this chapter we learned about a number of different strategies that one can use to help improve memory in everyday life. We now know that in order to benefit from using strategies we need to make a conscious effort to use them when faced with an appropriate situation. We also learned how we can apply these strategies to help us remember names, one of the most common complaints people have as they get older. Remember, the more you practice using these strategies, the easier and more effective they will become. You may not want to use all of them and they may not work perfectly the first time you try them, but with practice you will find the strategies that reliably work for you.

Let's now consider some examples to illustrate what we learned in this chapter.

- These strategies seem to take a lot of effort. Is it worth it?
  - For most people these strategies do take effort to learn and apply, but the effort will help you to remember the information.

In addition, over time, as you find the strategies that work best for you and continue to practice them, they will become easier. These strategies are an effective way to help improve your memory in everyday life.

- You've lost your car in a parking lot several times. Why does that happen and what can you do about it?
  - o One common reason for losing your car is that you were distracted when you parked and were not focused on where your car was. Pay active attention to where you are parking. Notice the signs and sights around you. Use visual imagery, rhyming, or another strategy to remember where you parked.
- Your wife says you have a "selective memory" because you forget the chores she tells you to do. Is there anything you can do to help yourself remember what she says?
  - o Often spouses tell you things, such as errands they want you to run, when you are distracted. Your wife may be telling you to pick up the laundry while you are watching the ball game or doing yard work. To remember what your spouse is telling you, eliminate or minimize distractions, practice active attention, and use repetition. So turn off the television, make eye contact, and repeat what she says.
- You're not a "visual" person, so you don't think visual imagery will work for you.
  - o Not every strategy is right for everyone. Some strategies work for some people and not for others. The best way to find out what works for you is to try each strategy several times and see what happens. Remember, don't give up if it doesn't work the first time, but if you're having trouble after several attempts, it may be that strategy isn't right for you. Most people can find several strategies that work well for them.
- I get so embarrassed when I can't remember someone's name that I've started avoiding some social situations.
  - o Trouble remembering names is one of the most common problems people have as they age. Try to relax by taking a couple of slow, deep breaths and remind yourself that difficulty with names is common. If possible, review the names of people you

are likely to encounter at your next social event ahead of time. Use some of the strategies you've learned to improve your ability to learn new names. If you can't recall someone's name, just be honest with them—they may also be having trouble remembering your name, and even if they aren't, chances are they know just how you're feeling!

18

Which Memory Aids Are Helpful?

There are many paper, mechanical, and electronic aids available to help us get organized and take the burden off of our memory. Some people are reluctant to use memory aids, saying, "I've never had to use a calendar before and I don't want to now," or "I've never needed a pillbox; I've got my own system." Other people worry that their brain will get lazy if they use these types of aids. The truth is that if you know someone with an excellent memory, chances are that person uses memory aids—you should, too.

THE THREE GOLDEN RULES

We begin with three golden rules to follow when using these types of aids:

Rule 1: Don't delay. To successfully keep track of things with memory aids, don't delay. For example, if your alarm goes off to remind you to take your medication, stop what you are doing and take your medication. Write down appointments immediately.

Rule 2: Keep it simple. Avoid redundancy. For example, instead of having four calendars, use just one. Simplicity reduces confusion.

Rule 3: Make it routine. Use your memory aid all the time, every time. Once you are in the habit of using the aid, you will use it automatically, even when you are tired, rushed, or distracted.

GET ORGANIZED

Jack and his daughter, Sara, are out for lunch. Jack is struggling with his memory for a number of things, such as remembering errands and groceries. Because his memory was quite good in the past, he had always relied on it and never used memory aids before.

"Sara, can you help me remember that I need to pick up bread, cold cuts, and cheese on the way home?" Jack asks. "Speaking of memory, I don't know how you can keep track of everything you need to do for work plus your family schedule, grocery lists, shopping lists, and other stuff."

"Dad, most people don't memorize all of those things in their head," Sara chuckles as she pulls out a piece of paper and a pen from her purse and writes down "bread," "cold cuts," and "cheese." "I use lists and other systems to help me remember. I'll show you when we get home."

It turns out that individuals who have never been good at remembering tend to have an easier time with memory loss than those who have had an excellent memory all of their lives. The reason is that those who have never been good at remembering developed organized systems and used aids when they were younger—systems and aids such as those described in this chapter. As their memory began to worsen, they simply relied more upon the aids that they were already using. It is harder for those who always relied upon their previously excellent memory to develop new systems and routines. The bottom line is that if you already use these types of aids, great, keep using them! If you haven't tried them yet, now is the time to get organized and give them a try.

DESIGNATE A MEMORY TABLE

"You know what the worst thing is," Jack begins as they are driving back to Sara's house. "I'm spending twenty minutes each morning looking for where I put my glasses, keys, and wallet the night before."

"That's easy to fix," Sara responds as she parks in her driveway. "Come on in and I'll show you." She opens the side door of her house. "When I arrive home each day, I put my keys, glasses, and purse right here on this table so I always know where they are if I need them, and they're ready for me to take when I go out the next day."

Do you ever find yourself scrambling to find your keys, cell phone, glasses, or other items as you prepare to leave your home? If so, consider placing a memory table (or bowl or basket) near the door. Commit to a routine that includes placing all items in this area when you come in the door so that you know where to find them when you are leaving the house. Over time you will begin putting the items there automatically, eliminating the need to search the house for what you need every time you are going out. One caveat: Make sure that your memory table doesn't become a clutter table. Place only those things that are important in this area, and regularly clean and organize the area to make sure other miscellaneous items don't accumulate. If the area becomes cluttered, it will not be effective.

USE A PILLBOX

Jack is also having trouble keeping track of whether he has taken his medications. "Now I've got pills for blood pressure, cholesterol, memory, plus those vitamins. I don't want to forget any of them, and I don't want to take them twice by accident."

Sara walks into the kitchen and says to Jack, "I use this pillbox here to keep track of my medications. On Sunday I fill it up, putting my morning pills in each of the 'AM' bins and my evening pills in each of the 'PM' bins. I keep it on the kitchen table so it's right here when I have breakfast in the morning and dinner at night. That way I never need to wonder whether I have taken my medications or not."

Do you ever have trouble remembering to take your medications? Are there times when you are not sure if you've taken your medications for the day or not? Using a pillbox to organize your medications can be extremely helpful. Pillboxes can help remind you to take your medications, help you remember if you've already taken them, and ensure you are taking the proper dose at the correct time. The first step is to choose a pillbox that works for you. There are numerous styles of pillboxes available today. Your basic pillbox has one compartment (that can be small or large) for each day of the week and comes in one-week, two-week, or one-month options. There are also pillboxes with separate compartments for twice-daily medications (morning and evening), or three-times-a-day medications (morning, afternoon, and evening). Pillboxes can have a variety of other options: color-coded compartments, Braille lettering, built-in alarms, display screens, and even communication devices that alert physicians or family members when medications are taken. It can be helpful to talk to your doctor when trying to decide which type of pillbox is best for you. Some providers may give you a free pillbox, and some insurance companies will cover the cost of your pillbox.

Once you've decided on a pillbox, the next step is to pick a day of the week or month when you will organize your medications from their containers into your pillbox. Sometimes people will choose to have a family member or professional do this task for them. Some pharmacies will do it for you, preparing a month's worth of medications in blister packs for a small additional fee. Figure out what pillbox system works best for you and stick with it.

RELY ON CALENDARS OR DAILY PLANNERS

"I see you have your calendar on the refrigerator," Jack remarks.

"Yes, that's our family calendar," Sara replies. "Everyone can add things to it, and we see it every time we are in the kitchen. Where do you keep yours?"

"In the basement."

"In the basement? But how often do you see it there?"

"Not very often, now that I think of it . . . I used to have it in the basement so that I would keep track of my different customers and their appointments before I left the house in the morning through the basement door into the garage. But I confess that now that I'm not working, I don't really look at it that often because it is in the basement . . . maybe I should move it to the kitchen."

Everyone can benefit from using a calendar or daily planner to keep track of appointments and important dates. If you don't already use a calendar, we recommend you start. Many people use calendars but don't take full advantage of them. Make sure your calendar is in a place where you see it daily.

When you use your calendar, it is important to be sure that you are noting all the important information you will need for each appointment. It can be helpful to think of the five "W"s when scheduling appointments in your calendar: WHEN, WHO, WHERE—and lastly—WHAT and WHAT. WHEN is the date and time of the appointment? WHO is the appointment with? WHERE is the location (and phone number) of the appointment? WHAT is the content of the appointment, and WHAT should you bring? For example, *Saturday, June 12, 3 PM; Becca Jones; 123 Main Street, Mayberry, 123–456–7890; Making desserts; Bring cookie cutters.* Or *Monday July 6, 10 AM; Dr. Harry Smith; 99 Pleasant Street, Everytown, 222–333–4444; Regular checkup; Bring insurance card and pill bottles.* Including all these bits of information makes it easier to remember to bring what you need, ask for directions, or call if you're running late.

If your calendar is kept at home, make sure it is placed in a visible, high-traffic location so you will see it on a regular basis. Look at your calendar each evening to see what you have coming up for the next day and week ahead. Review your calendar first thing in the morning so you know what your schedule is. If you keep your calendar at home, write down the day's appointments with all the information (or take a picture of your day with your phone). You can also use this time in the morning to set any alarms you will need to help remind you of appointments later in the day.

TAKE ADVANTAGE OF TECHNOLOGY

"There's no doubt that it would make it easier for you to see your calendar every day if it was in the kitchen," Sara agreed. "Another thing you could do is to use the calendar on your phone."

"There's a calendar on my phone?" Jack asks. "Wait, don't tell me, it's one of those 'apps,' right?"

"Exactly! The advantages of the calendar on your phone include that it is always with you, you can write as much information about the appointment as you like, and you can have alarms and reminders set up to make sure you won't forget about the appointment. That's what I do for work."

We could write a separate book on all of the technology that is available to help with thinking and memory. Smartphones have many features that can help you remember, including electronic calendars that will alert you of upcoming appointments and alarms that can be set to remind you of things like when to take your medications, when to make a phone call, or even when to leave the house to get to an appointment. They also have a notes section that you can use to write down things during the day that you don't want to forget. If you have both a cell phone and a home phone, you can also call your home phone and leave yourself a message of something you need to do when you get home. If you have Internet access, you can arrange to receive email alerts about all sorts of things, such as birthdays, anniversaries, and other important dates. These are just a few ways you can make use of technology, and there are many other smartphone applications and technological aids out there. Look around and talk to others to get ideas for what technology may be useful in your life.

KEEP A NOTEBOOK

Another way to keep track of information is to keep a paper notebook that you bring with you wherever you go. The best notebooks are those that fit in a pocket or purse so that you will be less likely to leave it behind. In your notebook you can keep track of appointments and things you need to do that day, grocery and other shopping lists you are making, and information people give you during the day that you need to remember. Once you get home you can transfer the important information to your calendar or daily planner.

MAKE LISTS

Jack, still looking at Sara's refrigerator, sees a partially completed grocery list on a long self-sticking note, along with several other notes, including "Remember to pick up a birthday card" and "Change the oil."

"I guess you don't keep everything you need to remember in your head . . ." Jack says half to Sara, half to himself.

If you don't already do so, making lists is an easy and useful way to remember information. Most people rely on grocery lists to remember what they need when shopping. To-do lists can also help you to stay on task and accomplish errands that need to get done. You might create a list of questions that you want to ask your doctor at your next visit and bring it along with you so you don't forget to discuss important topics. Keeping a pen and pad with you and making use of your smartphone applications are good ways to make sure you are always able to create a helpful list when needed.

USE REMINDER NOTES

Post-it™ and other reminder notes can help you remember numerous things in your daily life. Leave yourself a note on the door if there is something you need to bring with you the next day. Leave yourself a reminder note in the morning to remember to do something later in the day. You might stick the note "Defrost the chicken" on your refrigerator door before leaving for work in the morning so that you are reminded to take the chicken out of the freezer when you get home in the afternoon. As with our other techniques, there are multiple ways to use reminder notes. One important rule is to discard the note when the action has been completed so that you don't wind up with old notes everywhere. With some creative thinking you can figure out how best to incorporate reminder notes into your routine.

DEVELOP A ROUTINE

"That's right, Dad, I don't keep everything in my head," Sara agrees. "Between work, my daughter, and our complicated schedules, we need to use calendars, lists, reminders, and pillboxes to keep things straight. But the most important thing is that we have a routine of how we do things."

"What do you mean?" Jack asks.

"When I get home—as I was saying—I always put my keys, glasses, and purse on the hall table. I take my medications with breakfast and dinner. Everyone knows to add groceries to the shopping list on the refrigerator. And I always put new appointments right into my calendar . . . I've found if I wait and try to put them in later, I often forget parts of them—or even the whole appointment."

One useful way to improve your memory for regularly occurring events is to develop routines. When an activity becomes part of a well-established routine, you don't need to spend the same amount of mental energy required to remember the task. For example, if you have trouble remembering to take your morning medications, place them next to your coffee maker and make a routine of having your medications before you pour your first cup of coffee. For evening medications, placing them next to your toothbrush and taking them before you brush your teeth can become a routine. There are many other ways to use a daily, weekly, or monthly routine to your advantage. You can set aside one or two days of every month to pay your bills. You can even contact the services you pay bills to and request that all of your bills be due on the first of the month. Then set aside the last Saturday of every month to pay your bills. Think of other activities you need to remember in your own life that could become routines. To start a new routine, it may help to write it out. Over time these activities will become habit, and you will do them automatically.

MEMORY AIDS ARE FOR EVERYONE

Jack thought about Sara's words. He had felt it was "admitting defeat"—that his poor memory had "beat" him somehow—if he decided to give in and use a pillbox or rely upon a calendar. He was relieved to find out that even his smart, organized daughter with a great memory still found these kinds of memory aids useful.

You don't need to have a problem with your memory to benefit from the aids discussed in this chapter. Anyone of any age can keep track of more information by getting organized and using memory tables, pillboxes, calendars, smartphones, notebooks, lists, reminder notes, and routines.

SUMMARY

Memory aids can be pencil and paper or can take advantage of smartphone apps, electronic pillboxes, and other rapidly advancing technology. If you are feeling reluctant to try or rely on memory aids, keep in mind that the people you know who seem to have the best memories likely use these types of aids.

Let's now consider some examples to illustrate what we learned in this chapter.

- You have a key hook by your front door, but you still end up misplacing your keys. Often you find them on the counter or in your pocket. What's going on?
  - o Remember an important Golden Rule: Make it routine! Many of these memory aids need to be used consciously at first; over time they will become automatic. For example, if you have installed a key hook—good for you—that is the first step. The next step is to make sure you are very consciously using your new aid— the hook to hang your keys on—every time. Without conscious effort we often fall back into old habits—like throwing our keys on the counter or leaving them in our pockets. After several weeks or months of consciously using your new aid, you will begin to use it automatically, even when you are not thinking about it.
- You have a calendar at home that you update at the end of the day with any new appointments, but you find that you are still missing appointments that never made it on to the calendar. Why?
  - o Remember the first Golden Rule: Don't delay! If you have appointments that you are making throughout the day but you're waiting until the evening to write them down, you may forget them (or get them mixed up) by the time evening comes. Make sure you are using your memory aids right away, when information is fresh. It may be helpful to have a pocket calendar, notebook, or other aid you carry on your person to write down appointments in the moment and then later transfer them to a larger household calendar.
- Your pillbox is on the kitchen table. You have no difficulty taking your medications at breakfast and dinner. But even though you are home, you just can't seem to remember to take your two o'clock meds.
  - o Because morning and evening routines are fairly regular, it is easy to make taking medications a part of these routines. In the middle of the day, however, your schedule likely varies, and it can be more difficult to create a routine. In these cases it can be

helpful to always have your afternoon medications on your person and use an aid—such as an alarm on your watch or phone—to remind you to take your medications.

- You've never had to rely on a calendar or notes before and are feeling a little embarrassed about using them now. Shouldn't you just be able to "try harder" to remember things?
  - o The changes that occur in the brains of healthy, normally aging individuals can make it more difficult to remember information. Even if you were once able to remember all your appointments, errands, social events, and other information without a calendar or other aid, that may not be the case now. In addition, most well-organized middle-aged and even young adults use these types of aids. There is no reason to be embarrassed about using memory aids—it's a skill most highly accomplished individuals use daily.

Step 7

PLAN YOUR FUTURE

In Steps 1 through 6 we learned how to tell if your memory is normal, what the common causes of memory loss are, how to treat memory loss with medications, what diet to follow and exercises to do to stay mentally healthy, and how to improve your memory performance by engaging in strategies, using memory aids, and being social engaged. In this last step we will discuss how to plan your future proactively. We'll tackle thorny issues such as the use of guns and power tools, the legal matters that should be attended to, and whether there need to be changes in working and driving. We'll also discuss some of the positive things that you can do to improve your life and that of the next generation.

19

Will Changes in My Memory Change My Life?

Do you have to stop driving if you are diagnosed with a memory disorder? Can you continue managing your financial affairs? Should you give away your guns and power tools? Do you have to stop working? Should you move out of your home? These are some of the more common—and important—questions that are raised when we make a diagnosis of a memory disorder. The goal of this book is to help you stay independent and not let memory problems interfere with your doing everything you want to in life. But how do you balance your independence with your safety and that of others? We explore these and related questions in this chapter.

GET HELP FROM FAMILY OR FRIENDS WHEN INVESTING AND MANAGING MONEY

Jack received a notice in the mail a few weeks ago that his retirement plan is changing and he needs to choose which fund he is going to put his life's savings in. He has all the different options laid out on his kitchen table. He's not sure which fund to choose. He calls his daughter, Sara, to ask if she can stop by to give him some advice.

"Thanks Sara," Jack says when she arrives. "I really appreciate your helping me with this financial stuff. I just want to make sure I don't make any dumb decisions."

"It's no problem, Dad," Sara responds. "This stuff is pretty complicated for anyone."

Even the most intelligent individuals with perfect memory will sometimes make poor investment decisions leading to significant financial losses. Investing is a complicated art and depends upon awareness of, and memory for, some of the most recent information along with good judgment, reasoning abilities, and a bit of luck. Given the complexity of investing, it is not surprising that many individuals who eventually developed a memory disorder made poor investment decisions in the years prior to their diagnosis. The tragedy is that sometimes lifelong savings or retirement funds are lost within a short period of time. If you are having memory problems for any reason, we recommend that you pursue investing and other financial matters with someone you trust, such as a family member, close friend, or financial advisor with whom you have worked before. Note that we are not suggesting that you turn all of the decisions over to that person—just that you allow them to be part of the process. Similarly, it is a good idea to have someone look over your checkbook and bill paying periodically to make sure that no errors are creeping in and no one is taking advantage of you.

AVOID TELEMARKETERS

A related issue is telemarketers—those annoying individuals who call you on the phone trying to get you to buy something, donate money to some cause, or sign up for a new credit card. Make sure that all of your phone numbers are registered on the National Do Not Call Registry. Unfortunately, the registry doesn't stop all unwanted calls. You might consider purchasing a phone with caller ID so that you will know who is calling. Don't answer the phone if you don't recognize the number. Set your cell phone up to "silence unknown callers." If you miss a call from a real person you want to speak with, you can always check your messages and call them back. Lastly, as you know, you should never give a credit card number or banking information over the phone or by email.

INVITE A FAMILY MEMBER OR FRIEND TO GO FOR A DRIVE

After they finish going over the financial stuff, Sara gets ready to go home.

"Now don't forget, we're meeting the attorney tomorrow," she says as she is leaving. "Why don't you pick me up at work and we'll drive there in one car. I've written the appointment, the attorney's address, and my new work address in your calendar on the refrigerator."

The next day Jack copies down the appointment time along with the attorney's name and address into his new pocket notebook. He also copies down Sara's new work address. He knows the part of town where it is located, although he has never been to her new office. It should only take him twenty minutes. He pulls out of the driveway and heads to her office.

As he is driving, things don't look quite familiar. He realizes that some of his old landmarks aren't there anymore. *Where's the old Sears building?* Jack asks himself.

Twenty minutes have gone by. Jack cannot find Sara's new office building. He pulls over to the side of the road, puts the car in park, and pulls out his cell phone. "Sara, I'm having trouble finding your office. . . . Yes, I'm on Main Street, but I couldn't find the Sears building to know where to turn." Sara gives Jack directions, and he's back on track. He arrives a few minutes later and Sara, waiting on the curb, hops into the passenger seat.

Sara was surprised that her father had trouble finding her office, even though he hadn't been there before. *He used to know this city like the back of his hand,* she thinks to herself. "Dad, have you had any trouble driving?" she asks.

"Only a bit with directions, like now. I haven't had any 'fender benders' or anything like that."

Sara watches her father's driving closely as they travel to the attorney's office. He's driving an appropriate speed, using his turning signals correctly, seeing and stopping for pedestrians crossing in the middle of the street where they aren't supposed to. She feels perfectly safe and comfortable with his driving.

There are two basic types of difficulty that you may experience while driving. The first is getting lost. Although it is inconvenient, we don't worry too much about your getting lost. If you get lost, you can always pull over and ask for directions, click on an app in your smartphone, grab a paper map from your glove compartment, or call someone for directions. The second difficulty is that someone may not be a safe driver. Whether the problem is driving too fast or too slow, not seeing or stopping for pedestrians or red lights, or driving on the wrong side of the road, if someone isn't a safe driver, they should not drive.

How do you know if you are a safe driver? Well, it may seem like a silly question—obviously you wouldn't keep driving if you weren't driving safely, right? Turns out when it comes to driving, people are not good judges of themselves. If you have been diagnosed with any type of memory disorder, it is best to invite a family member or a friend to go for a drive with you monthly along whatever route you typically drive just to make sure you are still a safe driver. Make it fun—go out for dinner or a cup of coffee. Studies suggest that your children—assuming they are now adults—make the best driving observers.

What happens if you disagree with your family—they think you shouldn't drive but you believe you are driving just fine? In that case we recommend that you have a formal driving evaluation. Some states offer these evaluations through the Department of Motor Vehicles. Rehabilitation hospitals offer driving programs that will not only evaluate your driving but also help you to become a better driver. Some of these programs may cost a few hundred dollars, but they are well worth it—less expensive than a single accident.

The Hartford Foundation has created a number of helpful publications related to driving safety and cognitive decline that can be downloaded for free. These publications include information to help increase understanding of how cognitive changes might influence driving safety, assist in planning for potential changes in future driving status, and support you if you need to stop driving now or in the future. Many other organizations, such as the Alzheimer's Association, have similar resources. See Further Reading for details.

TAKE CARE OF LEGAL MATTERS NOW

Jack and Sara arrive on time at the attorney's office.

"How can I help you today," the attorney asks.

"My doctor diagnosed me with this 'mild cognitive impairment,'" Jack explains. "It's not too bad right now, but it may get worse in the future. So, my doctor said that now is the best time for me to make sure that I have all the paperwork signed that I might need in the future."

"I can help you with those things," responds the attorney. "We can go over your decisions today and get everything signed next week."

Whether or not you have been diagnosed with a memory disorder, now is a great time to get those legal papers in order. Be proactive—don't wait for a crisis to occur. In addition to a regular will, we recommend you have the following documents:

- **A living will** indicates the medical choices you would wish to make if you are unable to make them, such as whether you would want attempts to be made to restart your heart if it were to stop beating.
- **Power of attorney** is the document that allows you to name an individual to make legal and financial decisions if you are unable to make them for yourself.
- **Power of attorney for healthcare** is the document that allows you to name an individual to make medical and other healthcare decisions if you are unable to make them for yourself. Such decisions might involve choosing between different physicians and other healthcare providers; different long-term care facilities; and different types of treatment (for example, surgical versus medical treatment for cancer).

GIVE AWAY GUNS AND POWER TOOLS

Now that Jack's memory is a bit better on the medication that his doctor prescribed and—with Sara's help—he's more organized and better able to compensate for his memory with his calendar, notebook, reminders, to-do lists, and routines, he doesn't want to want to sit home all day. He would like to work part time. Having worked as an electrician most of his life, he begins looking for work in construction. Things have changed a bit, however, at the construction site. Now the foreman wants them to memorize safety rules and a series of checks to do for each tool every time they use it. Jack realizes that this job may not be the best one for him.

Safety is important not only on the road but also in the home. Guns and power tools represent two of the biggest hazards for anyone, regardless of age or memory. If you are having trouble with your memory, however, those hazards become much more dangerous. We know of individuals who have lost fingers from power tools and one terrible incident when a safety catch was unintentionally turned off on a gun. So, if you are having trouble with your memory, we recommend that you give away your guns and power tools. Your local police department will be happy to take in your guns, and we're sure that you can find a friend or relative to give the power tools to.

FIND THE RIGHT JOB

Jack is continuing his pottery class. After class one day Jack asks his teacher if she knows of anyone looking for part-time help.

"Actually," replies the teacher, "We're looking for someone to help out part time in our shop."

Jack looks pleased but puzzled. "I didn't think my pottery was good enough to sell in a shop," he says.

"Well," the teacher begins with a small smile, "that might be true, but the help we need is with other things. We have enough people making pottery, but we need help in the storeroom, packing up the pottery in boxes for shipping, and waiting on some of the customers when we get busy. There will always be one of us around to answer questions. I've seen how hard you work and how good you are with people."

"OK," Jack says, "that actually sounds great; it's just what I'm looking for. I just need to tell you one thing. I've seen my doctor about my memory. She says I've got this 'mild cognitive impairment.' I don't think it should interfere with my working in the shop, but I just wanted to let you know before you hired me."

"As it turns out," the teacher responds, "I know all about mild cognitive impairment. My father had it as well, and he did just fine for many years. If you want the job, it's yours."

Should you continue working if you have been diagnosed with a memory disorder? The answer depends on a few things, including whether you want to work, what your job is, and how long you have been doing the work. In general, working is always good, and so if you can continue to do your job well and safely, we would recommend that you do so. Working provides a healthy daily routine, intellectual stimulation, and social opportunities. It can also help with your mood and self-esteem. To reap these benefits, it doesn't matter if the job is paid or volunteer.

Good jobs to continue (or start) are those that involve making things without the use of power tools, including crafts, artwork, flower arranging, and knitting. Working in any type of a store where you can go at your own pace and there is someone around to ask questions is another example of a good job.

Jobs that are not good include those that involve supervision at almost any level, such as watching children at a daycare center or managing a business. Other jobs that are not good are those that involve memory, judgment, and reasoning and those that directly affect people's lives, such as a clinical or legal profession.

TALK TO FRIENDS AND FAMILY ABOUT YOUR MEMORY

Jack is having lunch with his friend Sam at his local community lodge.
"I've been thinking a lot about our conversation the last time we were here at the lodge a few months ago," Jack begins.
"The one when I told you that I thought you should get your memory checked out?" asks Sam. "I wasn't sure if you were going to thank me—or hit me."
"I wasn't sure myself," Jack says, chuckling. "I wanted to tell you that I did see my doctor about my memory problems, and I am sure glad that I did. She diagnosed me with this 'mild cognitive impairment' and has me on treatment for both Alzheimer's and strokes."
"I'm so sorry to hear about your diagnosis . . ."

"I'm not—I knew I was having memory problems, but I thought it was part of getting older and that nothing could be done about it. Now I know what's going on and I'm on a medication to help. So I wanted to thank you, Sam, for saying something. Even though we've been friends a long time, I'm sure it must have been difficult for you to do so."

"Yes, but after everything that I've been through with my wife, Mary, I know how important it is to jump on memory problems early," explains Sam.

OK, so you have some memory problems. You've confided in your spouse, child, or close friend who is right there to support you. But what about others? Should you mention your memory problems to your boss, coworkers, tennis partner, book club, or bridge group? This question does not have one right answer. It depends upon a number of factors, including how well you know the person, how supportive they are likely to be, and how likely your memory problems will become noticeable during your time with the person. Much of the answer, therefore, depends on how well your memory is doing. One general comment: it is our experience that most people wait too long to tell their family and friends.

Let's consider the following scenario. No one has noticed your very mild memory problems but you. You have recently been diagnosed with mild cognitive impairment and started on the medication donepezil (brand name Aricept) that can turn back the clock on your memory problems for six to twelve months. In this case you should have about six to twelve months in which no one will likely notice your memory problems. That doesn't mean that you should keep it a secret, but you probably can if you want to. After that time, it is likely that others will begin to notice some of the minor problems that you have noticed. That would be the time to tell most people you are friends with. So at that time, when you're playing tennis with an acquaintance, go ahead and ask her to help you keep track of the score, explaining that your memory isn't what it used to be.

Here is another scenario. This time it is one of your friends who asks if there is anything wrong with your memory. You go and get it checked out. You are told you have the beginnings of Alzheimer's disease and are started on donepezil. Can you keep it a secret? Because some people have already noticed your memory problems enough to say something to you, it is likely others have noticed as well. Don't be afraid—confide in your friends now, and tell them that you are having trouble with your memory. Good friends will be supportive.

GET THE SUPPORT YOU NEED TO STAY IN YOUR HOME IF YOU WISH

"How is Mary?" asks Jack.

"Well, her Alzheimer's is pretty bad now," Sam says. "She's in a memory care facility where they specialize in people who have advanced dementia like her."

"When did she move?"

"About six months ago. I was able to help her and keep up with everything until she started having a lot of accidents, and then it just became too much for me. But it's OK. She's in a great place, it is close by, and I visit her every day."

"I'm glad she's in a good place," Jack says. "I guess I might be following her . . ."

"Oh, I wouldn't worry about that anytime soon," Sam says quickly. "It was about eight years from the time that Mary's memory problems were as mild as yours until she moved into the facility."

If you have been diagnosed with a memory disorder, you might be wondering if you will need to move out of your home and into a facility. The short answer is that if you have been reading this book, your memory problems are likely mild enough that you can remain right in your home for a number of years. Over time, you may need more help from family, friends, or others. Listed below are some of the services that are available to make it easier for you stay in your home.

- **Meals on Wheels** provides prepared meals delivered to your door.
- **Visiting nurses** can give you medications and help with other medical issues such as checking your blood pressure or blood sugar if you have diabetes.
- **Homemakers** come to the house to help with laundry, cooking, light cleaning, and similar tasks.
- **Home health aides** can help with any personal care activities that you are having trouble with, such as bathing.

Talk to your doctor if you are interested in these home services or contact the Alzheimer's Association for more information. In addition, every day there are more retirement communities opening up that create a wonderful community in addition to providing assistance should you need it in the future— everything from a nurse stopping by daily dispensing medications to a specialized memory care facility. Assisted living and long-term care facilities are other options. Note that Medicare pays for some in-home services and Medicaid pays for some long-term care. Assisted living and retirement communities are generally self-pay, although in some states (such as Vermont) Medicaid pays for assisted living.

SUMMARY

There are a few life changes that are important to make if you are having memory problems. Give away guns and power tools. Take advice from family and friends when it comes to investing, managing money, and deciding if you should have a driving evaluation. Find a paid or volunteer job that you enjoy and that memory issues won't interfere with. Talk with friends and family about your memory so that they can understand and be supportive. Make sure your living situation is right for you and get help if you need it. Lastly, everyone should have legal documents such as a living will and power of attorney in place now—don't wait for a crisis to occur.

Let's now consider some examples to illustrate what we learned in this chapter.

- You have been successfully managing your retirement portfolio on your own for many years. Why should you ask your family to help just because your doctor says you have mild cognitive impairment?
  o Investing is a complicated business that often requires keeping many different pieces of information in mind at once. If you are having difficulty remembering information—even a tiny bit— you might end up making a bad investment because you couldn't keep in mind all of the different factors. For this reason it is a good practice to go over your decisions with someone you trust before they are finalized.
- You have never had a problem driving until last week when you couldn't find a friend's house that you have been driving to for many years. Does this incident mean you should stop driving?
  o Not necessarily. Having difficulty finding an address—or even getting lost—doesn't mean that your driving isn't safe. Invite a friend or family member—one of your grown-up children is best—to go for a drive with you. If he or she feels that you are a safe driver, then you can work on mapping out a route so you can drive back to your friend's house.
- Your children never thought you were a safe driver and will tell you that right now without stepping into the car. You've never had an accident and you think you are a good driver. You've just been diagnosed with a memory disorder. What should you do?
  o You should get a driving evaluation at either the Department of Motor Vehicles in your state or at a rehabilitation hospital. Even if it costs a few hundred dollars, that is less than the cost of a single accident. (And if you pass the test, you can tell your children that they are wrong!)

- You've been working as a nurse dispensing medications for more than fifty years. Even though you've been diagnosed with a memory disorder, you still know more than all of the new nursing graduates coming in put together. Do you need to stop working?
  - Yes and no. Because memory problems could lead to you giving a patient the same medication twice or forgetting to give a medication, it is important to stop that part of your job. Luckily, there is a lot more to nursing than dispensing medications, so there are many parts of nursing you would have no trouble doing. Speak to your supervisor about how your job could be altered so you could do it safely.

20

Where Do I Go from Here?

So now you've done it all: you've figured out if the changes you've noticed in your memory are related to normal aging or not. You received advice and perhaps tests and medications from your doctor. You're eating right, exercising regularly, and getting a good night's sleep. You are using different strategies and aids to keep your memory performance optimal. And you've made any changes needed in your driving, working, investing, and other issues. Where do you go from here? In this last chapter we'll discuss some of the positive, proactive things that you can do regardless of the cause of the changes in your memory.

GET SUPPORT FROM FAMILY AND FRIENDS

"How are you feeling?" John asks Sue as they are driving to the memory center. Sue is going to have her memory retested now that she is sleeping better and has had time to work on her anxiety and depression with physical exercise, yoga, and the medication prescribed by the neurologist.

"I feel great. Although I know my memory isn't perfect, I feel so much better about it now. And those memory strategies that I learned actually work—now I know what to do when I really need to remember something."

They arrive at the memory center. To their surprise, they see their friends Mary and Sam in the waiting room talking with some others there.

Sam looks up as Sue and John enter the room. "Hi, Sue, hi, John . . . I didn't expect to see you here at the memory center."

"Well," Sue responds, "I followed your advice and—rather than just worrying about it—I got my memory checked out!"

"We're here for Mary's follow-up appointment," Sam says, as he looks over at the man he was speaking with before. "Let me introduce you to my friend Jack and his daughter, Sara."

"So he told you, too, that you should get your memory checked out," Jack says to Sue as they all introduce themselves.

"Yes," Sue responds, "and I'm glad he did. I was so worried about my memory it was making me sad and anxious—which only made my memory worse!"

"Yeah, I confess I wasn't happy to hear Sam tell me that he thought my memory was going, but I'm also glad that he did."

Having concerns about or problems with your memory is hard, but it is even more difficult without your friends and family there to support you. Enlist your spouse, your children, or a close friend to confide in and share your concerns. Don't be alone worrying about your memory.

PARTICIPATE IN RESEARCH

"Jack was just telling me he's going to participate in some research," Sam says.

"Yup, I'm looking forward to helping out," Jack explains.

"I'm hoping that this new, experimental medication will help your memory, Dad," Sara adds.

"Well, that would be great and I hope so, too," Jack agrees. "But I'm doing it so that by the time you're my age—or maybe your daughter is—we won't have to worry about memory and Alzheimer's, because we'll have a cure."

There are many different types of memory research that you can participate in whether your memory is normal or you have a memory disorder. Clinical trials of new medications can lead the way toward a cure for memory disorders. Diagnostic clinical trials evaluate new methods to diagnose memory disorders, such as using electroencephalography (EEG), MRI, or a simple blood test. There is also research evaluating new strategies to improve memory, the best physical exercise to do, and the best foods to eat. If you can imagine it, there is probably a study out there to evaluate it. Most research studies are carried out in the clinic or hospital, although in some studies the researcher can come to your home or do the study virtually over video. Whatever the setting or goal, participating in research is one way to turn your memory problems into a very positive way you can give back to others and the next generation.

A great place to start finding out about research opportunities in your community is through the Alzheimer's Disease Research Centers funded by the National Institutes of Health (www.nia.nih.gov/health/alzheimers-disease-research-cent ers). These centers conduct all of the different types of research we described, including clinical trials. Check the website to see if there is a center close to you. Another place to get information about clinical trials going on in your area is to contact Trial Match at the Alzheimer's Association (https://trialma tch.alz.org). You can also go to https://clinicaltrials.gov/ and type in appropriate keywords such as "mild cognitive impairment," "Alzheimer's disease," or "Lewy body."

VOLUNTEER WITH ADVOCACY AND SUPPORT ORGANIZATIONS

Sue is called from the waiting room to have her pencil-and-paper testing.

"Good luck," John says.

Sue smiles. She feels a confidence about her memory that she hasn't had in a long time.

Thirty minutes later Sue and John are sitting in the neuropsychologist's office.

"I have some good news for you," she says. "You scored in the normal range on all of our tests."

"Does that mean my memory is normal?"

"Yes—and it means the memory difficulties that you were having before were likely due to the combination of side effects from the sleeping medications you were taking, the low level of your thyroid hormone, vitamin deficiencies, a bit more alcohol than we recommend—and the depression and anxiety you were experiencing."

Sue and John share a smile with each other.

On the drive home, Sue says to John, "I'd like to work helping others with their memory. I'd like to share some of what I learned about all the different things that can cause memory problems, and let people know about the importance of sleep, exercise, yoga, and getting your memory checked out."

"And don't forget all those strategies you learned," John adds.

"Yes, them, too . . . I think I'm going to find a good place to volunteer where I can help with all of those things and more. People need to know that they shouldn't ignore concerns about their memory—there's so much today that can be done to help."

John smiles.

Get involved. Volunteer. Work with others. Help increase awareness and decrease the stigma related to memory loss, Alzheimer's disease, and dementia. Raise money for research.

Share what you have learned. Volunteer for an information or crisis hotline. Lobby local and national politicians. There are many advocacy and support organizations that would benefit from your energy, enthusiasm, and commitment. The Alzheimer's Association is one such organization; there are also many other local, national, and international organizations that you can join. Search the web to find one nearby or perhaps a national or international one that best fits your interests.

GET MORE INFORMATION

There are many places you can turn to for additional information. At the end of this book in the Further Reading section you will find some relevant resources.

TAKE CONTROL OF YOUR MEMORY

Jack and Sara are driving home from their appointment. Jack is unusually quiet.

"What are you thinking about?" asks Sara.

"I'm thinking about all this memory stuff," Jack responds. "I feel so much better now that I know what is going on with my memory and that I'm on the right medicine. Using the calendar, memory table, and lists are working out great, and even the diet you've got me on isn't so bad."

"That's great to hear, Dad. I'm glad that you're feeling better about your memory after getting it checked out."

"Yes, and I'm very grateful to Sam for saying something to me and starting me down this path. I've just been thinking of one of our hockey buddies . . . he has been having trouble remembering what days we are playing, where we are practicing. . . . Now that I know more about memory problems and Alzheimer's and strokes, I bet that his memory isn't right. When I get home, I'm going to find him and tell him he should get his memory checked out!"

Don't let concerns about your memory become overwhelming. Don't wait for memory problems to be disabling. Don't be passive when it comes to your memory. Be proactive. If, after reading this book, you are concerned about your memory, get it checked out. Have the courage to find out if something is wrong. As we have described, there is much that can be done to help improve your memory regardless of what your memory problems are due to. Medications to help your memory work best when started early. You may also find out that nothing is wrong, that the changes in memory you have experienced are part of normal aging, or are something that can be easily treated such as a vitamin deficiency or a hormone imbalance. See your doctor. Use the information in this book. Get a good night's rest. Make changes in your diet. Start exercising regularly. Use strategies and memory aids to improve your day-to-day memory abilities. Take control of your memory.

SUMMARY

Memory problems are not something to hide from or ignore. Be proactive. With support from your family and friends, you will be in a good position to work with your doctor and address your concerns about your memory. Whether your memory is normal or not, participating in research is one way to help us find a cure for memory disorders, so that there will be even more treatments available for your children and grandchildren. Volunteering with organizations dedicated to helping people with memory disorders is another way to give back and share what you have learned. There are also many resources you can use to get more information about memory disorders, from both government agencies and private organizations.

Let's now consider some examples to illustrate what we learned in this chapter.

- You're concerned about your memory, and, after reading this book, you are sure that you are going to be diagnosed with Alzheimer's disease. Is there any benefit to seeing your doctor?
  - o Yes, for a number of good reasons. First, it might not be Alzheimer's disease. Your memory problems might be due to a vitamin deficiency, hormone imbalance, sleep disorder, depression, anxiety, or even normal aging. Second, if you are diagnosed with Alzheimer's, the medications that are used to treat it work best when started early. Lastly, there are new medications being developed in clinical trials that you could qualify for if your memory disorder is detected early enough.
- You would like to help further the research toward finding a cure for memory problems, but your memory is normal. Is there any research that you can participate in?
  - o Yes, absolutely! There are many research opportunities for those who are aging normally. Most studies that aim to develop a new diagnostic test, strategy, diet, or exercise for those with memory problems need healthy older adults, too. There are even clinical trials for individuals with concerns about their memory who perform normally on cognitive tests. See the Further Reading section to learn how you can participate.
- You've finished reading this book and you continue to have concerns about your memory. You're a private person and wouldn't usually share information about your health with anyone. Should you share your concerns with a family member or close friend?
  - o Yes, for several reasons. You can ask your friend or family member whether she or he has noticed any slippage of your memory. If you do go to see your doctor to get your memory problems checked out, it can be helpful to have another pair of eyes and ears so that you won't miss anything that the doctor is saying. Lastly, it can be lonely and anxiety-provoking to worry about memory problems by yourself; it's much better to share concerns with someone close to you.

Appendix

MEDICATIONS THAT CAN
IMPAIR MEMORY

Note that it is important to consult your doctor prior to stopping or lowering the dose of one of your medications. In addition, some medications must be lowered slowly or complications, such as seizures, may occur.

Anticholinergic Antidepressants

Most currently prescribed antidepressants are safe with few side effects. The ones that do cause memory problems are those that are anticholinergic. Acetylcholine is an important chemical in the brain that is necessary for normal memory function. Medications that are anticholinergic disrupt the activity of this important brain chemical, impairing memory and sometimes causing drowsiness and confusion as well. Older antidepressants with prominent anticholinergic side effects include the following:

- Amitriptyline (Elavil, Endep)
- Amoxapine (Asendin)
- Clomipramine (Anafranil)
- Desipramine (Norpramin, Pertofrane)
- Doxepin (Adapin, Sinequan)

- Imipramine (Tofranil)
- Mirtazapine (Remeron)
- Nortriptyline (Pamelor, Aventyl)
- Paroxetine (Paxil)
- Protriptyline (Vivactil)
- Trazodone (Desyrel)
- Trimipramine (Surmontil)

Antihistamines

Because they contain older formulations of antihistamines, many allergy medications, cold and flu remedies, nighttime pain relievers, and over-the-counter sleeping pills impair memory and cause drowsiness and confusion. Some of the older antihistamines that may impair memory include the following:

- Brompheniramine (Lodrane)
- Chlorpheniramine (Chlor-Trimeton, others)
- Diphenhydramine (Benadryl, others)
- Doxylamine (Unisom, others)
- Hydroxyzine (Vistaril, others)

Antipsychotics

Antipsychotics are medications that have been developed to treat young adults with schizophrenia or mania, although they are often prescribed for individuals with dementia with difficult behaviors. Memory impairment is common with these medications, particularly the older, so-called typical antipsychotics:

- Chlorpromazine (Thorazine)
- Fluphenazine (Prolixin)
- Haloperidol (Haldol)
- Loxapine (Adasuve)
- Mesoridazine (Serentil)

- Molindone (Moban)
- Perphenazine (Trilafon)
- Thioridazine (Mellaril)
- Thiothixene (Navane)
- Trifluoperazine (Stelazine)

The newer, "atypical" antipsychotics listed here are less likely to cause memory impairment, although they absolutely still can, particularly in high doses:

- Aripiprazole (Abilify)
- Asenapine (Saphris, Sycrest)
- Brexpiprazole (Rexulti)
- Cariprazine (Reagila)
- Clozapine (Clozaril)
- Iloperidone (Fanapt)
- Lurasidone (Latuda)
- Olanzapine (Zyprexa)
- Paliperidone (Invega)
- Pimavanserin (Nuplazid)
- Quetiapine (Seroquel)
- Risperidone (Risperdal)
- Ziprasidone (Geodon)

Anxiety Medications: Benzodiazepines

Benzodiazepines are one class of medications used to treat anxiety that almost always causes memory impairment, drowsiness, and confusion. In fact, when doctors perform a medical procedure but don't want you to remember it (such as a colonoscopy), this is the class of medication they give you. Note that any reduction or stopping of these medications should always be done under the supervision of your doctor; seizures may occur if they are stopped abruptly. Some commonly prescribed benzodiazepines, all of which cause memory impairment, are as follows:

- Alprazolam (Xanax)
- Chlordiazepoxide (Librium)
- Clobazam (Onfi)
- Clonazepam (Klonopin)
- Clorazepate (Tranxene)
- Diazepam (Valium)
- Estazolam (Prosom)
- Flurazepam (Dalmane, Dalmadorm)
- Lorazepam (Ativan)
- Nitrazepam (Mogadon)
- Oxazepam (Serax)
- Temazepam (Restoril)
- Triazolam (Halcion)

Dizziness and Vertigo Medications

If you experience dizziness, nausea, and vertigo due to an inner ear infection or being on a boat, it is fine to take one of these medications for a day or two if it makes you more comfortable. But you don't want to take the medications on this list for more than that, as they are either anticholinergic, antihistamines, or benzodiazepines, which (as described earlier in this appendix) all cause memory impairment:

- Clonazepam (Klonopin) (benzodiazepine)
- Diazepam (Valium) (benzodiazepine)
- Dimenhydrinate (Dramamine) (anticholinergic)
- Lorazepam (Ativan) (benzodiazepine)
- Meclizine (Antivert, Vertin) (anticholinergic)
- Metoclopramide (Reglan)
- Promethazine (Phenadoz, Phenergan, Promethegan) (antihistamine)
- Scopolamine (also known as hyoscine, anticholinergic)

Herbal Remedies

Herbal remedies are just another type of medication with their own side effects; they are not intrinsically safer just because they are herbal. Common herbal medications and their major side effects include the following:

- Ephedra (ma huang): insomnia, nervousness, tremor, headache, seizure, high blood pressure, heart problems, strokes, kidney stones; memory may or may not be affected.
- Ginkgo biloba: bleeding (Note: There is no evidence that ginkgo biloba improves memory, and we do not recommend its use.)
- Kava: memory impairment, sedation, confusion, abnormal movements
- St. John's wort: memory impairment, fatigue, dizziness, confusion, dry mouth, stomach upset

Incontinence Medications: Antispasmodics

Bladder incontinence leading to urinary accidents is a serious problem that may make it difficult for people to go out in public and may result in wearing adult absorbent undergarments. If you have incontinence, are taking one of these medications, and it is working to stop or greatly diminish urinary accidents, we recommend continuing it. However, many people take incontinence medications without a noticeable improvement. If this is the case, and it is one of the anticholinergic medications listed here, we recommend speaking with your doctor to see if it can be reduced, eliminated, or substituted for one that works as well (or better) with fewer side effects:

- Darifenacin (Enablex)
- Fesoterodine (Toviaz)
- Flavoxate (Urispas)
- Oxybutynin (Ditropan)
- Solifenacin (Vesicare)
- Tolterodine (Detrol)
- Trospium (Sanctura) (may have relatively fewer side effects)

Migraine Medications

Not all migraine medications cause memory impairment, but some do. If you are frequently taking one of the medications on this list, consider speaking with your doctor about trying a migraine medication that is less likely to cause memory impairment.

Anticholinergic Antidepressants

- Amitriptyline (Elavil, Endep)
- Doxepin (Adapin, Sinequan)
- Imipramine (Tofranil)
- Nortriptyline (Pamelor, Aventyl)
- Protriptyline (Vivactil)

Butalbital-Containing Medications

- Butalbital–acetaminophen–caffeine (Fioricet, Vanatol LQ, Vanatol S, Esgic, Capacet, and Zebutal)
- Butalbital–aspirin–caffeine (Fiorinal)

Narcotics

- Codeine–acetaminophen (Tylenol–Codeine #3), oxycodone–acetaminophen (Percocet)

Seizure Medications

- Topiramate (Topamax)
- Divalproex sodium (valproic acid and sodium valproate) (Depakote)
- Gabapentin (Neurontin)

Muscle Relaxants

Medications to treat muscle spasms may be effective, but they many also cause memory impairment, drowsiness, and confusion, which these do:

- Baclofen (Lioresal)
- Carisoprodol (Soma)
- Chlorzoxazone (Lorzone)
- Cyclobenzaprine (Flexeril)
- Metaxalone (Skelaxin) (may have relatively fewer side effects)
- Methocarbamol (Robaxin) (may have relatively fewer side effects)
- Orphenadrine (Norflex) (anticholinergic)
- Oxazepam (Serax) (benzodiazepine)
- Tizanidine (Zanaflex)

Narcotics: Opioids

Sometimes narcotic pain medications are needed. By itself, pain will impair memory. However, narcotics should only be used for brief periods of time. Studies have shown that they tend not to work for chronic pain, cause memory impairment and confusion, and are quite addictive. Narcotics likely to cause memory impairment include the following:

- Alfentanil
- Buprenorphine (Belbuca, Probuphine, Buprenex)
- Codeine (in Tylenol–Codeine #3 and some cough syrups)
- Fentanyl (Actiq, Duragesic, Fentora, Abstral, Onsolis)
- Hydrocodone (Hysingla, Zohydro, in Vicodin, Lorcet, others)
- Hydromorphone (Dilaudid, Exalgo)
- Levorphanol (Levo-Dromoran)
- Meperidine (Demerol)
- Methadone (Dolophine, Methadose)
- Morphine (MS Contin, Kadian, Morphabond)
- Nalbuphine (Nalbuphine)
- Opium
- Oxycodone (OxyContin, Oxaydo in Percocet, Roxicet)
- Oxymorphone (Opana)
- Pentazocine (Talwin)
- Propoxyphene (Darvon)
- Remifentanil (Ultiva)
- Sufentanil (Dsuvia, Sufenta)

- Tapentadol (Nucynta)
- Tramadol (ConZip, Ultram)

Nausea, Stomach, and Bowel Medications

Most gastrointestinal medications do not cause memory problems, but the ones listed here do:

- Chlordiazepoxide (Librium) (benzodiazepine)
- Clidinium (Librax) (anticholinergic)
- Dicyclomine (Bentyl) (anticholinergic)
- Diphenhydramine (Benadryl, others) (antihistamine)
- Glycopyrrolate (Cuvposa, Glycate, Robinul) (anticholinergic)
- Haloperidol (Haldol) (antipsychotic)
- Hyoscyamine (also known as scopolamine) (Levsin, Hyosyne, Oscimin) (anticholinergic)
- Lorazepam (Ativan) (benzodiazepine)
- Methylscopolamine (Extendryl, AlleRx, Rescon, Pamine) (anticholinergic)
- Metoclopramide (Reglan)
- Prochlorperazine (Compro) (antipsychotic)
- Propantheline (Pro-Banthine) (anticholinergic)

Seizure Medications: Anticonvulsants

Anticonvulsants are prescribed not only for seizures but also for nerve pain, peripheral neuropathy, headaches, mood stabilization, and agitation. Some of the anticonvulsants that can cause memory impairment include the following:

- Clobazam (Onfi) (benzodiazepine)
- Clonazepam (Klonopin) (benzodiazepine)
- Diazepam (Valium) (benzodiazepine)
- Divalproex sodium (Depakote)
- Gabapentin (Neurontin) (side effects may be tolerable when used in low doses [100 to 300 mg per day])
- Lorazepam (Ativan) (benzodiazepine)
- Nitrazepam (Mogadon) (benzodiazepine)

- Phenobarbital
- Phenytoin (Dilantin)
- Pregabalin (Lyrica)
- Primidone (Mysoline)
- Sodium valproate (Depakote)
- Tiagabine (Gabitril)
- Topiramate (Trokendi, Qudexy, Topamax)
- Valproic acid (Depakote)
- Vigabatrin (Sabril)

Sleep Medications

Melatonin and acetaminophen are two medications that can sometimes be helpful for sleep. Otherwise, we recommend non-pharmacological treatments for sleep problems. Medications used for sleep problems that are likely to cause memory impairment and confusion the next day include the following:

- Amitriptyline (Elavil, Endep) (antidepressants)
- Clonazepam (Klonopin) (benzodiazepine)
- Diphenhydramine (Benadryl, in Advil PM, Tylenol PM, others) (see the earlier section on "Antihistamines")
- Doxepin (Adapin, Sinequan) (anticholinergic antidepressant)
- Estazolam (Prosom) (benzodiazepine)
- Eszopiclone (Lunesta) (similar to benzodiazepines)
- Flurazepam (Dalmane, Dalmadorm) (benzodiazepine)
- Gabapentin (Neurontin) (anticonvulsant)
- Lorazepam (Ativan) (benzodiazepine)
- Mirtazapine (Remeron) (anticholinergic antidepressant)
- Quetiapine (Seroquel) (antipsychotic)
- Ramelteon (Rozerem) (similar to benzodiazepines)
- Suvorexant (Belsomra) (similar to benzodiazepines)
- Temazepam (Restoril) (benzodiazepine)
- Trazodone (Desyrel) (anticholinergic antidepressant)
- Triazolam (Halcion) (benzodiazepine)
- Zaleplon (Sonata) (similar to benzodiazepines)
- Zolpidem (Ambien, ZolpiMist) (similar to benzodiazepines)

Tremor Medications

Tremor medications likely to cause memory impairment, drowsiness, and confusion include the following:

- Benztropine (Cogentin) (anticholinergic)
- Hyoscyamine (Levsin, Hyosyne, Oscimin) (anticholinergic)
- Primidone (Mysoline) (anticonvulsant)
- Trihexyphenidyl (Artane) (anticholinergic)

Glossary

Note: These definitions are accurate for how these terms pertain to memory, memory loss, and the disorders of aging as discussed in this book; they are not intended to be general definitions. The step and chapter numbers in parentheses indicate where these topics are discussed in more detail.

AD8: An eight-item questionnaire that can be completed by individuals concerned about their memory or, more commonly, someone close to them, such as a family member. (Step 2, Chapter 4).

Aducanumab: A drug (brand name Aduhelm) administered monthly by intravenous infusion that is a monoclonal antibody designed to remove amyloid plaques from the brain. Whether it produces benefit to patients is unclear. Many patients experience side effects of brain swelling or bleeding. (Step 4, Chapter 11)

Aduhelm: See *Aducanumab*.

Alcohol-related dementia: Alcohol can cause permanent damage to the brain leading to dementia in two main ways. When intoxicated, individuals are more likely to experience head trauma that can damage the brain, due to either falling down or getting into physical fights. These trauma-related head injuries often damage the frontal lobes, leading to problems with disinhibition (see *Frontal lobes*). The second way is when alcohol use is combined with nutritional deficiencies, specifically of thiamine (Vitamin

B1). This combination can lead to degeneration of several parts of the memory circuit (mammillary bodies and anterior nucleus of the thalamus), leading to permanent and sometimes profound amnesia. Individuals at risk for alcohol-related dementia should take thiamine daily.

Alzheimer's disease: A disorder of the brain caused by two brain abnormalities, amyloid plaques and neurofibrillary tangles. Symptoms typically begin with memory loss. When thinking and memory are impaired but function is normal, we refer to it as mild cognitive impairment due to Alzheimer's disease. When day-to-day function is impaired, we refer to it as Alzheimer's disease dementia. (Steps 2 and 3)

Amyloid PET scan: See *PET scan.*

Amyloid plaque: Microscopic collections of beta-amyloid, parts of brain cells, as well as other substances that are found between and outside brain cells. Beta-amyloid is an abnormal protein that collects in Alzheimer's disease. (Step 3, Chapter 8)

Amyotrophic lateral sclerosis (ALS): A degenerative disease that affects motor function, involving the upper and lower extremities and ultimately all muscles in the head, leading to difficulty speaking, swallowing, breathing, and death. It is sometimes seen with *frontotemporal dementia.*

APOE-e4 gene: A gene that increases the probability that a person will develop Alzheimer's disease. (Step 3, Chapter 8)

Aricept: See *Cholinesterase inhibitor.*

Beta amyloid: See *Amyloid plaque.*

Cat scan: See *CT scan.*

Cerebral amyloid angiopathy: When amyloid accumulates in the walls of small blood vessels in the brain. It can lead to bleeds which are usually small but sometimes large.

Cerebrovascular disease: See *Stroke.*

Cholinesterase inhibitor: Medications that improve memory by inhibiting the breakdown of the chemical acetylcholine, an important neurotransmitter in the brain. Donepezil (brand name,

Aricept), rivastigmine (brand name, Exelon), and galantamine are three commonly used cholinesterase inhibitors to treat memory disorders, including Alzheimer's disease. (Step 4, Chapter 11)

Chronic traumatic encephalopathy: A progressive disorder of thinking, memory, mood, and behavior caused by multiple violent blows to the head, such as commonly occurs in boxing and football. (Step 3, Chapter 6)

Clinical trial: Research studies of new medications to either improve cognitive function or slow the decline of a brain disease. In most trials some people get the new medication and some people receive a placebo, with the assignment being random. (Step 4, Chapter 11)

Cognitive behavioral therapy: Typically short-term, goal-oriented psychotherapy using a practical approach to problem-solving. The goal is to change patterns of thinking and/or behavior which can, in turn, change the way people feel. (Step 4, Chapter 12)

Cognitive testing: See *Neuropsychological tests.*

Consolidation: The process by which new memories, initially formed by the hippocampus and related structures in the temporal lobe, become old memories stored in the cortex. Both rapid eye movement (REM) and non-REM sleep are important for consolidation. (Step 5, Chapter 13)

Cortex: The outer layer of the brain where consolidated memories are stored. (Step 2, Chapter 4)

Corticobasal degeneration: A degenerative disease affecting thinking, memory, behavior, and movement leading to *dementia.* Different than most other dementias is that it typically begins with asymmetric involvement of an arm or a leg, leading to loss of function in that limb. The limb starts by being clumsy, progresses to becoming useless, and finally stiff and difficult to move. Some individuals experience a jerky tremor, a limb that moves seemingly with a will of its own, behavior or personality changes, or effortful, nonfluent speech.

CT scan: A brain imaging study using X-rays that can show patterns of atrophy and strokes. (Step 2, Chapter 4)

CTE: See *Chronic traumatic encephalopathy.*

Dementia: When problems with thinking and memory reach the point at which independent function is impaired. (Step 3, Chapter 7)

Dementia with Lewy bodies: See *Lewy body disease.*

Diabetes: Diabetes can lead to memory loss and dementia in two main ways. When blood sugars are not well controlled, there may be an increase in *strokes* leading to *vascular dementia.* In addition, if blood sugars run too low (below the normal range), it can damage the *hippocampus,* the part of the brain that forms new memories.

Distorted memory: When a memory becomes changed or mixed up with another memory such that it is no longer accurate. (Step 1, Chapter 1)

Donepezil: See *Cholinesterase inhibitor.*

Exelon: See *Cholinesterase inhibitor.*

False memory: When we remember something that never happened. (Step 1, Chapter 1)

Frontal lobes: Located in the front part of your brain, just behind your forehead, the frontal lobes focus attention allowing us to efficiently store, retrieve, and organize our memories. (Step 1, Chapter 2)

Frontotemporal dementia: A degenerative brain disease that affects behavior first and foremost. Typically there are also problems related to thinking and memory, apathy or inertia, loss of sympathy or empathy, and abnormal eating behavior. (Step 3, Chapter 10)

Galantamine: See *Cholinesterase inhibitor.*

Hippocampus: The memory center of your brain, located on the inside and bottom of each temporal lobe, which are next to your temples on each side of your head, just behind your eyes. The left hippocampus is somewhat specialized for remembering verbal and factual information, and the right for nonverbal and emotional information. (Step 1, Chapter 1; Step 2, Chapter 3; Step 3, Chapter 8)

Human immunodeficiency virus (HIV)–associated neurocognitive disorder (HAND): HIV disease, alone or with opportunistic infections, can cause cognitive impairment and *dementia*. Common symptoms include difficulty processing information and performing complicated tasks. Memory problems can also occur, usually due to poor learning and impaired retrieval of information.

Lewy body disease/Lewy body dementia: A degenerative brain disease that has some combination of the following symptoms: features of Parkinson's disease, visual disturbances (including hallucinations), acting out dreams, and thinking and memory difficulties. (Step 3, Chapter 10)

Limbic-predominant age-related TDP-43 encephalopathy (LATE): A degenerative brain disease that causes symptoms similar to *Alzheimer's disease*. It is typically identified when Alzheimer's is suspected, but changes in beta-amyloid protein are not observed either in an *amyloid PET scan* or in spinal fluid from a *lumbar puncture*. (Step 3, Chapter 10)

Lumbar puncture: Commonly known as a spinal tap, a lumbar puncture is a procedure in which a small amount of spinal fluid is removed from the back. The fluid can be analyzed for beta-amyloid and tau, two proteins whose levels are abnormal in Alzheimer's disease. (Step 3, Chapter 8)

MCI: See *Mild cognitive impairment.*

Mediterranean diet: One of the few diets that may be beneficial for brain health. It includes fish, vegetables, olive oil, avocados, nuts, fruits, beans, and whole grains. (Step 5, Chapter 14)

Memantine: Available as generic and the brand, Namenda, memantine is FDA approved for the treatment of Alzheimer's disease for individuals in the moderate to severe stage of dementia. (Step 4, Chapter 11)

Mild cognitive impairment (MCI): A term used when a decline in memory or thinking (or both) has been noticed, impairment is present on tests of thinking and memory, but daily function is essentially normal. (Step 3, Chapter 7)

MRI scan: A brain-imaging study using magnets that can show patterns of atrophy and strokes. (Step 2, Chapter 4; Step 3, Chapter 6)

Multiple sclerosis (as a cause of dementia): A disease of the brain and spinal cord in which the myelin—the insulation around nerves—is disrupted by an autoimmune process. It typically presents with noticeable symptoms over hours or days, which may or may not resolve. Many individuals with multiple sclerosis never develop cognitive problems or dementia. When dementia does appear, it typically presents with slowed processing, inability to perform complicated activities, and easy or abnormal laughing and crying (*pseudobulbar affect*).

Namenda: See *Memantine.*

Neurofibrillary tangle: Parts of the skeleton and nutrient system of the dying brain cell which appear "tangled" under the microscope. These tangles form after the cell has been damaged by amyloid plaques or another process. (Step 3, Chapter 8)

Neurological exam: A specialized physical exam to evaluate the brain and nervous system. It includes testing vision, hearing, strength, sensation, movement, walking, and reflexes. (Step 3, Chapter 6)

Neurologist: A medical doctor who specializes in the diagnosis and treatment of disorders of the brain and other parts of the nervous system. (Step 3, Chapter 6)

Neuropsychological tests: Tests that evaluate different aspects of thinking and memory, which, in turn, help to determine how different parts of the brain are functioning. (Step 2, Chapter 5)

Neuropsychologist: A psychologist who has received advanced training in the use and interpretation of pencil-and-paper tests and questionnaires to help diagnose brain disorders and provide practical advice. (Step 2, Chapter 5)

Normal pressure hydrocephalus: A brain disorder caused by excess fluid in the brain, leading to a slowing of walking with small steps, an urgency to run to the bathroom to urinate, and poor attention, thinking, and memory. (Step 3, Chapter 10)

Parietal lobes: Parts of the brain that are important for attention and spatial functioning; they are affected early in the course of Alzheimer's disease. (Step 3, Chapter 8)

Parkinson's disease: A degenerative brain disease causing some combination of slowness of movement; slow, shuffling walking; and a tremor. Other symptoms can include loss of smell, constipation, and REM sleep behavior disorder. It may be treated by medications.

PET scan: A positron emission tomography (PET) scan is like an "inside-out" X-ray. With an X-ray, the radiation beams go from the transmitter, through the body, and collect on a film or X-ray detector. With an *amyloid* or *tau* PET scan, the radiation is built into a tiny molecule that is engineered to stick to either amyloid plaques or tau tangles. The molecule is injected through an intravenous (IV) catheter in the arm, and if there are any amyloid plaques or tau tangles in the brain, it will stick to them. The radiation of the molecule sticking to the plaques or tangles is then detected on the X-ray detector. (Step 3, Chapter 8)

Plaque: See *Amyloid plaque.*

Posterior cortical atrophy: Although not a disease in itself, it is a useful way to describe individuals with *dementia* who have visual problems as their most prominent symptom, while their other cognitive functions (such as memory, language, and behavior) are more or less intact. The name comes from the fact that the back or posterior part of the brain is most affected. (Step 3, Chapter 10)

Primary age-related tauopathy (PART): A degenerative disease in which *tau neurofibrillary tangles* develop in the *temporal lobes* leading to slowness of cognition and difficulty performing complicated tasks. It is not thought to lead to *dementia.* (Step 3, Chapter 10)

Primary progressive aphasia: A degenerative brain disease that affects language first and foremost. (Step 3, Chapter 10)

Progressive supranuclear palsy (PSP): A degenerative brain disease affecting thinking, memory, behavior, function, balance, speech, and eye movements. Individuals often begin with a slowing of eye movements and difficulty walking due to poor balance. They typically progress to difficulty looking down, frequent falls, speech difficulties, and swallowing problems, in addition to impairment in thinking, memory, and behavior.

Pseudobulbar affect: A disorder common in *dementia* in which individuals may laugh or cry with little or no provocation. Treatment is available.

Rapid forgetting: Even when information has been learned well, it is quickly forgotten, often leading to repeating questions and leaving important items unattended, such as leaving the stove on. (Step 2, Chapter 3)

Rivastigmine: See *Cholinesterase inhibitor*.

Screening test: A brief test of thinking and memory that can be used to detect cognitive problems, even if no symptoms are present. (Step 2, Chapters 4 and 5)

Small-vessel disease: See *Stroke*.

Spinal tap: See *Lumbar puncture*.

Stroke: Stroke occurs when an artery sending blood from the heart to the brain becomes blocked off; that part of the brain doesn't receive enough blood and dies. Because the problem is related to blood vessels, strokes are often called "vascular disease" or sometimes "cerebrovascular disease" to emphasize the problem is with blood vessels of the brain or "cerebrum." Small-vessel disease strokes from the blockage of small and microscopic arteries in the brain are typically silent and only detected on CT or MRI scans. (Step 3, Chapter 9)

Subjective cognitive decline: A term used when a decline in thinking and/or memory has been noticed by the individual and it is of sufficient concern to bring it to the attention of a doctor but tests of thinking and memory are normal as is daily function. (Step 3, Chapter 7)

Subjective cognitive impairment: See *Subjective cognitive decline*.

Tangle: See *Neurofibrillary tangle*.

Tau: A protein that is part of the skeleton and nutrient system of the brain cells. See also *Neurofibrillary tangle*. (Step 3, Chapter 8)

Tau PET scan: See *PET scan*.

Temporal lobe: See *Hippocampus*.

Thyroid: A gland in the neck that produces thyroid hormone. Abnormal thyroid hormone levels may cause impaired memory, difficulty concentrating, irritability, mood instability, restlessness, and confusion. (Step 3, Chapter 6)

Vascular cognitive impairment: Cognitive impairment due to stroke. (Step 3, Chapter 9)

Vascular dementia: Dementia due to stroke. (Step 3, Chapter 9)

Vascular disease: See *Stroke*.

Vitamin B$_{12}$: Deficiency of vitamin B$_{12}$ can cause serious problems with thinking, memory, and mood. Some individuals are unable to absorb B$_{12}$ even if their dietary intake is normal. (Step 3, Chapter 6; Step 5, Chapter 14)

Vitamin D: Deficiency of vitamin D has been associated with a higher risk of dementia, in general, and Alzheimer's disease, in particular. (Step 3, Chapter 6; Step 5, Chapter 14)

Further Reading

Note: Although extensive literature was reviewed to assure the most accurate and up-to-date medical and scientific content, only books, websites, and other reference materials accessible to a general audience have been included in this section. All those interested in the full list of sources used for this book may contact the authors, who will be glad to provide the full reference list.

BOOKS

Budson, A. E., & Kensinger, E. A. (2023). *Why we forget and how to remember better: The science behind memory*. New York: Oxford University Press.

• This book provides a detailed explanation as to how your memory works, as discussed in Steps 1, 2, and 5, as well as how to use that information to remember better, as discussed in Step 6.

Schacter, D. L. (1997). *Searching for memory: The brain, the mind, and the past*. New York: Basic Books.

• This book provides a wonderful overview of memory, with an emphasis on how false memories develop.

Schacter, D. L. (2021). *The seven sins of memory updated edition: How the mind forgets and remembers*. Boston: Mariner Books.

• This book provided much of the scientific content for Chapter 1.

NEWSPAPER, MAGAZINE, JOURNAL, AND ONLINE ARTICLES

The Alzheimer's Association Facts and Figures, http://www.alz.org/facts/overview.asp

• The document on this website, updated yearly, provided some of the clinical and scientific content for Chapters 4 and 8.

The scientific data, reviews, and interpretations that led to the FDA approval of aducanumab (Aduhelm) (Step 4, Chapter 11) may be found on this website:

• https://www.accessdata.fda.gov/drugsatfda_docs/nda/2021/761178Orig1s000TOC.cfm

A review of the some of the side effects of aducanumab (Aduhelm) (Step 4, Chapter 11) can be found in the following paper:

• Salloway, S., Chalkias, S., Barkhof, F., Burkett, P., Barakos, J., Purcell, D., Suhy, J., Forrestal, F., Tian, Y., Umans, K., Wang, G., Singhal, P., Budd Haeberlein, S., & Smirnakis, K. (2022). Amyloid-related imaging abnormalities in two Phase 3 studies evaluating aducanumab in patients with early Alzheimer disease. *JAMA Neurology, 79*(1), 13–21. https://doi.org/10.1001/jamaneurol.2021.4161

All of the following articles are related to the controversy regarding the brain-training industry discussed in Step 6, Chapter 16:

Cookson, C. (2014, October 26). The silver economy: Brain training fired up by hard evidence. Retrieved from http://www.ft.com/intl/cms/s/0/c6028b80-3385-11e4-ba62-00144feabdc0.html#axzz3yXpv8PMZ

Federal Trade Commission. (2016, January 5). Lumosity to pay $2 million to settle FTC deceptive advertising charges for its "brain training" program: Company claimed program would sharpen performance in everyday life and protect against cognitive decline. Retrieved from https://www.ftc.gov/news-events/press-releases/2016/01/lumosity-pay-2-million-settle-ftc-deceptive-advertising-charges

Federal Trade Commission. (2015, April 9). FTC approves final order barring company from making unsubstantiated claims related to products' "brain training" capabilities. Retrieved from https://www.ftc.gov/news-events/press-releases/2015/04/ftc-approves-final-order-barring-company-making-unsubstantiated

Max Planck Institute for Human Development and Stanford Center on Longevity. (2016, January 27). A consensus on the brain training industry from the scientific community. Retrieved from http://longevity3.stanford.edu/blog/2014/10/15/the-consensus-on-the-brain-training-industry-from-the-scientific-community-2/

Simons, D. J., Boot, W. R., Charness, N., Gathercole, S. E., Chabris, C. F., Hambrick, D. Z., & Stine-Morrow, E. A. (2016). Do "brain-training" programs work? *Psychological Science in the Public Interest: A Journal of the American Psychological Society, 17*(3), 103–186. https://doi.org/10.1177/1529100616661983

USEFUL WEBSITES

General Information

The National Institute on Aging, part of the National Institutes of Health, has a number of resources on their website: www.nia.nih.gov/alzheimers/publication/understanding-memory-loss/introduction. The Alzheimer's Disease Research Centers also provide information about memory loss including community talks and presentations: www.nia.nih.gov/alzheimers/alzheimers-disease-research-centers. If you have a scientific background and would like to find out about the latest research discoveries, you will find them all at the Alzforum: www.alzforum.org. The Alzheimer's Association is a nonprofit organization dedicated to providing the public with information and assistance in managing memory loss and dementia from any cause, not just Alzheimer's disease. You can start with their main website (www.alz.org) or find your local chapter here: http://alz.org/apps/findus.asp. You might want to join their mailing list so you can stay abreast of new developments and offerings. They have a 24/7 helpline offering information and advice in over 200 languages. They also offer support groups and educational sessions, online message boards, help finding research opportunities to become involved in, and information materials on numerous dementia-related topics. The Alzheimer's Society plays a similar role in England, Wales, and Northern Ireland (www.alzheimers.org.uk/), as does the Alzheimer Society in Canada (http://www.alzheimer. ca/) and Dementia Australia in Australia (https://www.dementia. org.au/).

AD8 Questionnaire

https://www.alz.org/media/Documents/ad8-dementia-screen ing.pdf

Body-Mass Index Calculator

https://www.nhlbi.nih.gov/health/educational/lose_wt/BMI/bmic alc.htm

Fish Mercury Levels

https://www.fda.gov/food/consumers/advice-about-eating-fish

For Clinical Trials

For Trial Match at the Alzheimer's Association: https://trialmatch. alz.org/, email trialmatch@alz.org, or phone 800-272-3900
For trials through the National Institutes of Health: https://clinica ltrials.gov/. Type in appropriate keywords, such as "mild cognitive impairment," "Alzheimer's disease," or "Lewy body."

For Driving

https://www.thehartford.com/resources/mature-market-excellence/ publications-on-aging
http://www.alz.org/care/alzheimers-dementia-and-driving.asp

For Help in the Home

https://www.alz.org/care/alzheimers-dementia-in-home-health.asp

Mindfulness and Meditation

https://nccih.nih.gov/health/meditation/overview.htm

Relaxation Therapy

https://nccih.nih.gov/health/stress/relaxation.htm

About the Authors

Andrew E. Budson received his bachelor's degree at Haverford College, where he majored in both chemistry and philosophy. After graduating cum laude from Harvard Medical School, he was an intern in internal medicine at Brigham and Women's Hospital. He then attended the Harvard-Longwood Neurology Residency Program, for which he was chosen to be chief resident in his senior year. He next pursued a fellowship in behavioral neurology and dementia at Brigham and Women's Hospital, after which he joined the neurology department there. He participated in numerous clinical trials of new drugs to treat Alzheimer's disease in his role as the Associate Medical Director of Clinical Trials for Alzheimer's Disease at Brigham and Women's Hospital. Following his clinical training he spent three years studying memory as a postdoctoral fellow in experimental psychology and cognitive neuroscience at Harvard University under Professor Daniel Schacter. After five years as Assistant Professor of Neurology at Harvard Medical School, he joined the faculty at Boston University in their Alzheimer's Disease Research Center as well as the Geriatric Research Education Clinical Center (GRECC) at the Bedford Veterans Affairs Hospital. During his five years at the Bedford GRECC, he served in several roles, including the Director of Outpatient Services, Associate Clinical Director, and later the overall GRECC Director. In 2010 he moved to the Veterans Affairs Boston Healthcare System, where he is currently the Associate Chief of Staff for Education, Chief of Cognitive & Behavioral Neurology, and Co-Director of the Center for Translational Cognitive Neuroscience. He is also the Director of Outreach, Recruitment, and Education at the Boston University Alzheimer's Disease Research Center, Professor of Neurology at Boston University School of Medicine, and Lecturer in Neurology at Harvard Medical School. Dr. Budson has had National Institutes of Health and other government research funding since 1998, receiving a National Research Service Award and a Career Development Award (K23) in addition to Research Project (R01) and VA Merit grants. He has given over 750 local, national, and international grand rounds and other academic talks, including at the Institute of Cognitive Neuroscience, Queen Square, London; Berlin, Germany; and Cambridge University, England. He has published eight books and over 125 papers in peer-reviewed journals, including *The New England Journal of Medicine*, *Brain*, and *Cortex*, and is a reviewer for more than fifty journals. He was awarded the Norman Geschwind Prize in Behavioral Neurology in 2008 and the Research Award in Geriatric Neurology in 2009, both from the American Academy of Neurology. His current research uses the techniques of experimental psychology and cognitive neuroscience to understand memory and memory distortions in patients with Alzheimer's disease and other neurological disorders. In his Memory Disorders Clinic at the Veterans Affairs Boston Healthcare System, he treats patients while teaching medical students, residents, and fellows. When not working or writing, he enjoys spending time with his family, traveling, running, skiing, kayaking, biking, and practicing yoga.

Maureen K. O'Connor graduated summa cum laude with a bachelor's degree from Ithaca College, where she majored in both psychology and religion. She received her doctorate in psychology from Indiana University of Pennsylvania, focusing her dissertation on the differentiation of depression versus Alzheimer's disease under the mentorship of Dr. David LaPorte. She attended Yale University School of Medicine for her predoctoral internship, where she conducted outpatient and inpatient memory evaluations for adults with a broad range of diagnostic presentations, including dementia, traumatic brain injury, and stroke. She went on to complete one year of postdoctoral residency at Cornell Weil Medical Center/Sloan Kettering Cancer Center and two additional years of residency at the Bedford Veterans Affairs Hospital/Boston University School of Medicine. In 2005 she accepted an appointment at the Bedford Veterans Affairs Hospital as the Director of Neuropsychology. In that role she established the Memory Diagnostic Clinic, specifically designed to evaluate and treat older Veterans with memory loss and to provide support to their families. In 2008 she was awarded board certification in neuropsychology by the American Board of Professional Psychology. In 2009 she accepted the Young Alumni Achievement Award from the College of Natural Sciences and Mathematics at Indiana University of Pennsylvania. She has served on the board of the Massachusetts Neuropsychological Society as the Chair of the Continuing Education Committee and the National Academy of Neuropsychology as the Chair of the Education Committee for. In 2019 she was appointed the Director of the Research Education Component at the Boston University Alzheimer's Disease Research Center. In 2014 she was promoted to the rank of Assistant Professor in the Department of Neurology at Boston University School of Medicine. Dr. O'Connor's research interests include understanding and developing interventions to improve the lives of adults with memory loss and the lives of the family members who help provide care. In 2005 she received a pilot grant from the Boston University Alzheimer's Disease Research Center to study the effect of exercise training on cognition. In 2006 she was the recipient of a New Investigator Research Grant from the National Alzheimer's Association designed to study the impact of caregiver training on managing neuropsychiatric symptoms in dementia. In 2014 she received a Research, Rehabilitation, and Development SPiRE Award to study the impact of an intervention designed to educate older adults about brain aging and dementia and lifestyle factors that contribute to brain aging. She is currently funded by the Alzheimer's Association and the National Institute of Aging to study dementia caregivers, their lived experiences, and interventions designed to provide them with support and skills training. In addition, Dr. O'Connor continues to evaluate and treat individuals with memory loss while teaching doctoral students, interns, and residents in neuropsychology. In her free time she enjoys running, cooking, and relaxing with her husband, their daughter, and their dog, Bruce.

Index

For the benefit of digital users, indexed terms that span two pages (e.g., 52–53) may, on occasion, appear on only one of those pages.
Tables are indicated by *t* following the page number